The Creative Dementia Practice Handbook

of related interest

Bridging the Creative Arts Therapies and Arts in Health
Toward Inspirational Practice
Edited by Donna Betts, PhD, ATR-BC and Val Huet, PhD
Foreword by Lord Alan Howarth
ISBN 978 1 78775 722 6
eISBN 978 1 78775 723 3

Drum Circles for Specific Population Groups
An Introduction to Drum Circles for Therapeutic and Educational Outcomes
Edited by Simon Faulker
ISBN 978 1 78775 524 6
eISBN 978 1 78775 525 3

Life Story Work with People with Dementia
Ordinary Lives, Extraordinary People
Edited by Polly Kaiser and Ruth Eley
Foreword by Joyce Dunne and Tommy Dunne
ISBN 978 1 84905 505 5
eISBN 978 0 85700 914 2

THE CREATIVE DEMENTIA PRACTICE HANDBOOK

Arts for Health and Wellbeing

EDITED BY

Maria Pasiecznik Parsons
and Richard Coaten

FOREWORD BY ALEXANDRA COULTER

Jessica Kingsley Publishers

London and Philadelphia

First published in Great Britain in 2026 by Jessica Kingsley Publishers
An imprint of John Murray Press

1

Contents

Section 3: Informing, Developing and Supporting

Foreword

Alexandra Coulter, *National Centre for Creative Health (NCCH)*

I am delighted to contribute a foreword to this important and timely publication. Maria Pasiecznik Parsons and Dr Richard Coaten are two of the most experienced and knowledgeable experts in the field of dementia and the arts and have drawn on the expertise of many others who feature in this practice handbook. The audience, as the title suggests, is primarily practitioners, particularly Community Practitioners and Creative Arts Therapists, who wish to advance their understanding and knowledge to inform their work. The handbook foregrounds the lived experience of people and values their voices while emphasising the central role of co-creation and person-centred approaches. Ronald Amanze says in Chapter 12:

> If it wasn't for art, I may have vanished by now. I know this as a fact. I would have disappeared. I would have become silent. I would never have been seen. I would have never been recognised as someone who had feelings and thoughts and aspirations. I would have been totally deleted from the radar by exclusion.

I will use 'creative health' as an overarching and inclusive term with a broad definition of the arts and creativity, from everyday creativity such as gardening or knitting at home to specialised arts practice across the range of artforms such as performing arts, literature and visual arts. Creative health can exist in homes, communities, cultural institutions and heritage sites or healthcare settings. It can contribute to the prevention of ill health, promotion of healthy behaviours, management of long-term conditions, and treatment and recovery across the life course. It can also encompass creative health approaches, for example co-production and creating change in how health services are delivered. This handbook will be of great interest not only to specialists working with people with dementia but also to many others working in the field of creative health. The content related to developing the workforce is highly relevant to the whole creative health workforce. Many creative health practitioners work with people with a range of health needs, one of which might be people living with dementia.

When we consider the subject of this handbook within the wider field of creative health policy, research and practice, it is notable that creative health with people living with dementia is one of the best established areas of practice and research. And within that, I think it would be uncontroversial to state that music and dementia has the highest profile in popular media, not least because of celebrity endorsement of activities such as dementia choirs. But as we see from this handbook, the practice extends across all artforms, and we read about the nuanced and layered ways in which different artforms can provide expression, solace and creativity when working with people with dementia.

The wider field is even more multifaceted and complex, within a matrix of different intersecting artforms, demographics, conditions and settings. This range and complexity can make it difficult to target decision makers with specific evidence and recommendations. In the National Centre for Creative Health's Creative Health Review, published in late 2023, the recommendations for government and metro mayors, with a clear ask for cross-governmental support. With the Labour Government's mission-led approach to policy, this cross-governmental approach becomes even more relevant and desirable. Not only does creative health sit between the established sectors of health and social care, and culture and the arts, it also plays a role in place-based approaches to community, in mitigating the negative social determinants of a lack of education, poverty and poor housing. Arguably, access to creativity and cultural opportunities is not only a human right but a social determinant in itself. To quote Professor Sir Michael Marmot:

> To reduce health inequalities, then, we need to create the conditions for the benefits of cultural and creative activities to spread to all members of society. It should form a key part of breaking the link between relative poverty and poor health. (NCCH and APPG AHW 2023 p.138)

Barriers to access to creativity and culture can be societal and systemic but can also be at the intimate and micro level. As we see in Chapter 3, 'A creative conversation about arts and memory', Jane's facilitation of John's access to his own creativity and engagement ranges from the practical, in providing materials and transport, to the subtle use of methods and strategies to prompt memory and recall.

Following Lord Darzi's independent investigation of the NHS in 2024, the government is developing a '10 Year Health Plan' with three priority shifts: to prevention, to community and to digital. Creative health plays an important role in prevention and population health. Creative health can support primary prevention in building social capital, social cohesion and improving wellbeing; and it can contribute to secondary and tertiary prevention in preventing, managing and treating specific conditions. For example, playing a musical instrument reduces cognitive decline and dementia, and gardening can lower blood pressure, reducing the risk of cardiovascular disease. In Chapter 16 on research and evaluation there is a full discussion of the wealth of research and evaluation studies that show the benefits of engagement in creative arts for people living with dementia.

There are many challenges to the ambition of integrating creative health more fully into health and care provision. Providing greater access to the benefits before people engage with health services, and helping to prevent people needing to access the beleaguered and overstretched NHS, are equally important and challenging. Health services as they are currently configured and funded in England are unsustainable in the face of ever-increasing needs and demands, and Lord Darzi's report recognised the fundamental change required. Creative health can play a dynamic role in this context. There are several references to systems thinking in the handbook. It is relevant at the individual level as highlighted in Chapter 13 on social prescribing, which identifies the complex context in which a person's needs may, or may not, result in a referral to an arts offer. It also provides a framework within which we can consider the role of creative health as a catalyst for change in health and care at scale. Change does not happen in a linear way as systems transition from old paradigms dominated by hierarchical structures and traditional medical models to emerging practices. 'Pockets of the future' can be found within the existing system (Systems Innovation Network). All of those reading this handbook can contribute to this collective endeavour and know that their contribution is valuable, part of a greater change to create a health and care system fit for the future and a healthy and health-creating society with people living healthier and happier lives.

References

NCCH and APPG AHW (National Centre for Creative Health and the All-Party Parliamentary Group on Arts, Health, and Wellbeing) (2023) *Creative Health Review: How Policy Can Embrace Creative Health.* https://ncch.org.uk/creative-health-review

Co-Editors' Preface

The roots of this handbook lie deep in our respective backgrounds: in professional social work, academia, social care leadership and management of Creative Dementia Arts Network (CDAN) (Maria) and dance/theatre studies, management training, community dance practice, hospital arts coordination, hospital/community-based arts therapy, dance and movement psychotherapy and doctoral-level research (Richard). For a great many years, we have been fostering the growth of what is often referred to as 'creative arts *for* dementia' or even 'creative dementia'.

There is no standardised definition of the field of practice in which practitioners engage with people living with dementia using creative arts. We use both phrases, whilst co-authors use a range of other descriptors. We also think the goals and activities relating to creative arts for dementia align well with those of creative health.

We both have an interest in training and professional development for Creative Arts Therapists (CATs) and Creative Practitioners (CPs), now Creative Health Practitioners (CHPs), who work with people living with dementia. Richard, a dance and movement psychotherapist, currently runs training and professional development in the UK and Europe. Maria developed FLOURISH, CDAN's flagship creative arts and dementia training course for CPs. FLOURISH was paused during the COVID-19 pandemic and is due to be relaunched in a blended format.

We began our collaboration at the first CDAN arts for dementia conference in 2011. This brought together arts, health and social care practitioners, managers and staff, academics, and people living with dementia and their carers. For almost a decade, these annual conferences offered:

- plenaries about research and development in the field of creative arts for dementia
- creative practice workshops led by experienced creative arts practitioners and cutting-edge creative arts projects
- information stands and networking opportunities.

For a moment, amid the enlivening, supportive and informative intermingling of artists and practitioners from all creative disciplines, Richard felt the isolation he experienced as a community dance worker disappear. It was replaced by a feeling of being part of a rich and evolving community of arts-based practice with people living with dementia. As conference evaluations showed, this alone was an important conference takeaway.

The other conference evaluation messages were about unmet needs. Conference participants (and other UK CPs we worked with) continued to express frustration about the dearth of comprehensive or universal high-quality peer support and supervision, and training and professional development opportunities for creative arts practitioners working with people living with dementia.

During post-pandemic reflections, we conceived of this handbook. We were proud of the way in which the arts and culture sector had reconfigured what they did to meet needs for social connection, meaningful occupation, joy and hope amongst vulnerable isolated individuals, groups and communities. We were also acutely aware of the continuing impact of COVID-19 on arts organisations and venues and particularly on the livelihoods of CHPs, many of them freelancers, whose work is in any case precarious.

Maria had assembled a draft FLOURISH textbook that accompanied CDAN's short flexible practice learning course. We recognised this as the cornerstone for:

- developing a guide to good practice in creative arts in dementia
- raising the profile of creative arts for dementia by presenting the work of CPs and CATs.

We consulted further with colleagues, practitioners and managers in arts, health and social care via online webinars about what they wanted to find in a handbook for best practice. The answer was: an awful lot! The list included an understanding of dementia, values in practice, examples of what best practice looks like, skills, practitioner self-care and signposts to resources...

So we asked a diverse group of 24 people to work with us on bringing these ideas together and presenting them clearly to a wide readership. The result is what we hope will be a well-used practice handbook, made richer by the exemplary contributions of our co-authors. We thank them enormously for collaborating with us to produce a legacy of learning about good practice that we hope improves and facilitates the expansion of creative arts for dementia and inspires present and future generations.

Introduction

As co-editors, we hope that the rich seams of knowledge, skills and experience that are woven throughout the handbook will prove useful to both new and experienced practitioners and for staff in arts, health and social care who use creative arts to engage with people living with dementia. Before we introduce its contents, this feels like the right place to state that there is so much more to say on every topic in the book. Nevertheless, the extensive references and resources provided will, we hope, be useful in furthering learning and study beyond the handbook.

We think it's helpful to 'locate' creative arts for dementia in the field of creative health. Creative health refers to creative activities that promote health and wellbeing and prevent ill health. This construct was ushered in by *Creative Health: The Arts for Health and Wellbeing* (APPG AHW 2017). This landmark report is referenced frequently in the handbook and is mandatory reading for everyone working in our field of practice.

The handbook provides a view of current practice, policy and research in creative arts for dementia. It illustrates the huge diversity of this field, not only in the creative arts themselves but also among our authors. They include people living with dementia, carers, friends, musicians, composers, a playwright, poets, creative arts practitioners, community music practitioners, CATs, dance and movement psychotherapists, a performance artist, an arts and health consultant, managers, researchers and academics. We have listed them here to make a point about the fluidity of the field of practice and terminology. We have not been prescriptive about the way our authors should write about what they do or how they refer to themselves, sometimes in terms of their professional training, for example as an arts therapist, or as an artist, or as a practitioner describing themselves by arts form or work setting, hence 'community music practitioner'.

Here is a glimpse of the chapters in the order in which they appear. Do let interest or curiosity be your guide in choosing how to read this book...

Section 1: Practising Well contains two chapters that together make up the cornerstone of the handbook.

Chapter 1 conceptualises and contextualises creativity, arts and dementia. At its heart is the importance of putting the person living with dementia *first* in any creative engagement. Chapter 2, its companion piece, reflects on good practice informed by person-centredness, personhood and the Creative Health Quality Framework (CHQF). These principles underpin good practice and can be used by practitioners and commissioners, amongst others, to assure the quality of their work.

Section 2: Creative Arts Practice is the heart of the handbook, providing a view of the breadth of the field: the diversity of practitioners and facilitators, what they do and where, in 11 chapters. Chapter 3 is made up of conversations between a poet and painter who is living with dementia, and his wife, who is his carer. They talk about how he has adapted his artistic practice to take account of cognitive impairment, and their shared experience of how creative arts has helped them navigate changes in their lives. Chapter 4 focuses on how musicians compose music with people living with young onset dementia and their carers who take part in a long-established touring music programme that brings them together with musicians and university music students. In Chapter 5, attention is paid to the embodied and relational practices of somatic dance with people living with Parkinson's and their carers, and the author provides insights into her development as 'an artful carer'. In Chapter 6, a poet co-creating poetry with people living with dementia explains the process she uses to plan and run her sessions. A different kind of writing follows in Chapter 7, which offers a rare view of a playwriting group comprising a person living with dementia, a university lecturer and a playwright, co-creating a play about the experience of dementia. In Chapter 8, a different story is told by a museum manager and her team who co-produced a novel museum app to prompt memory and reminiscence. It demonstrates how arts and cultural venues can digitalise museum resources to respond to the needs of local people living with dementia and their families. The app can be customised and has been co-produced for the Liverpool Yemeni community and is being used globally.

Chapters 9 and 10 about creative arts in group care settings – care homes and hospitals respectively – highlight the importance of creative arts for frail residents and patients. We also see challenges for CPs of negotiating work with busy staff working in hectic environments. Chapter 11, about the Moving Kinship project, describes pioneering performative work that uses an intersectional lens to understand the nature of support for family carers and formal caregivers. This extends to non-verbal ways of relating to the person living in a non-verbal world in the later stages of the condition when language skills decline. Language is also the focus of Chapter 12 in which a colleague and friend of a music producer, poet and dementia activist provides a platform and scaffolding that enables him to talk about how he is living his life post-stroke by figuratively climbing mountains of hope.

How might painting, music and poetry be socially prescribed? In Chapter 13, the manager and senior staff of a large arts organisation reflect on their experiences of collaborating on a local scheme for social prescribing of the arts and lessons learnt.

Section 3: Informing, Developing and Supporting begins with four interconnected chapters about the creative health workforce. It begins with Chapter 14 on the broad canvas of training and professional development, including a cameo piece about creative dementia arts training. This is followed in Chapter 15 by a review of self-care, support and reflective practice, all fundamental but often neglected by practitioners due to their limited resources, particularly those who are self-employed – the focus of Chapter 16. Chapter 17, the final chapter in this sequence, takes a deeper dive into the working lives of three freelancers: two practitioners and a consultant in arts, health and heritage, examining the rewards and challenges of their precarious work.

Richard was the instigator of Chapter 18, designed to provoke a debate about the roles and relationships of CATs and CPs and the case for closer collaboration. We consider how this change could take place through the lens of systems theory.

The final chapter offers food for thought. In many ways, the *future* of creative arts and dementia is *here now*. We see this in the form of increasing prevalence of dementia in the UK and across an increasingly uncertain world. The need for support not only for individuals but also for family carers is vital. Here, we revisit topics, issues and ideas that have emerged from various chapters. Alongside this, we offer our thoughts about what we need to address now for creative arts for dementia to flourish in all communities and a well-trained, ethically, socially and culturally diverse workforce is to be developed. Whilst in themselves creative arts cannot provide a cure for dementia, they can benefit the health and wellbeing of people living with dementia and family carers who engage in creativity through the medium of relationships with practitioners.

We hope this handbook will encourage students, early career practitioners and others contemplating using arts to work with people living with dementia to join what is a vibrant community of practice. We also hope it will be read by commissioners, managers and funders of creative arts for people living with dementia. Their support is needed, given that practices described in the handbook do not take place in a vacuum but are parts of what is intricate (and often disjointed) health and care provision for individuals and families. Whilst not a frontline service, creative arts can, with core investment, help reduce risks and meet many of the social and psychological needs of a growing population affected by dementia. This enables individuals, carers and communities to thrive.

So, if you feel a little burnt out or seek food for thought, if you need to be challenged or better informed about the changes taking place in what is a fast-growing field of practice, dip in and enjoy!

Reference

APPG AHW (All-Party Parliamentary Group on Arts, Health and Wellbeing) (2017) *Creative Health: The Arts for Health and Wellbeing*. https://ncch.org.uk/appg-ahw-inquiry-report

PRACTISING WELL

CHAPTER 1

Creativity in Arts, Health and Dementia

Maria Pasiecznik Parsons and Richard Coaten

Introduction

Give me myself and I will be me
Give me an ear and I will speak
Give me patience and I will relax
Give me music and my heart will dance
Give me joy and I will laugh

These are the first five lines of 'Give Me...I Will', a poem by Keith Oliver (2019) who is living with dementia. Here, he makes a simple but profound point about relationships. For it is what we – caregivers, friends, communities and society – give and do in response to Keith's requests that enable him to have agency and pleasure in life. Given the focus of this handbook, the last lines are particularly relevant for practitioners, therapists and others who facilitate creative arts and engage people living with dementia.

This chapter contextualises both creative arts and dementia, giving equal weight to both. We begin by setting out some of the different ways in which dementia is defined, highlighting points of contention about what has become a major public health issue in the UK and globally. Under the heading 'Dementia: an overview', we begin with the biomedical model of dementia. Despite its weaknesses, highlighted by substantial social and psychological critiques, it continues to influence public perception and research priorities.

However, its predominance in a major aspect of dementia care has been superseded by an enriched model of dementia. Developed by Tom Kitwood, researchers and practitioners, this model is one of a number of pioneering ideas that are recognised as best practice in dementia care. Personhood is a core concept: the importance of recognising and supporting people living with dementia in their full humanity by seeing the *person* with dementia. A person's experience of dementia arises not only from biomedical phenomena, such as their degree of neurological impairment and their physical health, but also from social and psychological factors such as their personal biography and day-to-day interactions with other people. All care is person-centred. Importantly, Kitwood refers to arts and creative activities as ways of maintaining personhood.

The absence of a cure or disease-modifying treatment and widespread adoption of person-centred approaches in health and social care gave rise to a plethora of psychosocial and 'non-pharmacological' approaches to supporting people living with dementia. These are geared towards inclusion, socialisation and promoting health and wellbeing. Increasingly, these involve participatory arts and cultural activities.

This development mirrors what was happening in the larger arts-for-health movement, and this chapter summarises its development, noting how evidence of its benefits hastened its progress and encouraged the growth of arts movements for other health conditions, including creative arts for dementia. The expansion of this field of practice was aided by challenging the notion of 'creative genius' as intellectual prowess, conceptualising creativity as inclusive of people living with dementia and highlighting inclusive approaches including co-creativity.

The latter half of this chapter focuses on creative arts in dementia – on purposeful and planned practices in which creative arts are used to improve individual health and wellbeing and support quality of life. This approach is reflected in how we define creative arts in dementia and the inclusion of diverse art forms used by Creative Health Practitioners to work with people living with dementia. We also consider the settings in which they work and how this work is funded. Our conclusion acknowledges the complexity of this field of practice and the contribution of creative arts to enabling people living with dementia to express themselves, as chronicled in the pages of this handbook.

Dementia: an overview

There is no unequivocal answer to the question: what is dementia? Indeed, 'There are strong, sometimes conflicting opinions about what dementia is among the public, professional and research communities and within communities and families' (Manthorpe and Iliffe 2016 p.4). We begin with the biomedical model, which continues to dominate public perceptions of dementia despite its focus on pathology and cognitive deficit.

Dementia is viewed as a syndrome, a range of disorders with different causes that are characterised by impairment of cognitive function including memory, speech and language, perception, and decision-making and cognitive skills. It is a terminal condition; over time people become frailer and more vulnerable to illness as all systems contingent on brain health are affected. Dementia is categorised biomedically in terms of types. Alzheimer's disease (Alzheimer's type dementia or ATD) is the most prevalent, followed by vascular type dementia (VTD), caused by mini strokes, and then mixed dementia (usually a combination of ATD and VTD). Some two in ten people diagnosed with Mild Cognitive Impairment (MCI) experience small cognitive changes; some develop dementia but many continue living independently (Alzheimer's Research UK 2024).

Most people who develop dementia are aged 80–84 years old (National Institute for Health and Care Excellence 2025). Dementia with Lewy bodies most often triggers early onset or young onset dementia that affects people aged 45–65 years old (Carter 2022). Most people with a diagnosis of Parkinson's do not go on to develop dementia, although about a third will, usually in the later stages of the illness (Dementia UK 2025).

Dementia is a major global public health issue. Risks of dementia are highest amongst people aged 80+ hence the increasing prevalence and incidence in ageing populations. Over 55 million people are living with dementia across the world (Long, Benoist and Weidner 2023). In the UK, an estimated 982,000 people are living with dementia, and by 2040, this population is forecasted to increase to 1.4 million (Alzheimer's Research UK 2024). Dementia prevalence will increase more rapidly amongst members of Black and Minority Ethnic (BAME) communities than amongst those in the White British community (APPG Dementia 2013). The incidence of dementia was found to be 20% higher, and onset occurred at an earlier age, amongst people with Black British backgrounds compared with South Asian and White British groups (Mukadam *et al.* 2022).

In the UK, the cornerstone of support for people living with dementia in the community is unpaid carers – including family members, such as partners and (most often) daughters – and depending on the severity of cognitive and/or physical impairment, individuals themselves. Most are unpaid carers, whose care is valued at £21.1 billion (Alzheimer's Society and Carnall Farrar 2024). A third of people with dementia live in care homes (Oung, Lobont and Curry 2024).

In line with national dementia plans and directives (Journal of Dementia Care 2024) General Practitioners (GPs) can assess people with memory problems, but most are referred to local memory clinics where they are assessed and diagnosed and, if appropriate, prescribed symptomatic drug treatments (Alzheimer's Society 2025). Advice for individuals and families is provided by GPs and memory clinics, who also signpost patients and families to local service providers, Dementia UK and the Alzheimer's Society.

Remodelling dementia: from the biomedical to the biopsychosocial

Psychiatrists first defined dementia as a biomedical problem in the 1900s and later classified it as an incurable terminal disease. The process of medicalising dementia included mandating psychiatrists to provide diagnosis, treatment and care for patients, reinforcing it as an individual problem rather than a societal one (Bond 2001). The biomedical model is widely considered reductionist. This is because it assumes all features of the condition can be reduced to biological causes and does not take sufficient account of the heterogeneity of the dementia syndrome, differing symptom profiles and their impact on diverse individuals (Camic *et al.* 2018). For example, whilst the ability to carry out specific Activities of Daily Living (ADLs) are compromised at different stages of dementia (Giebel *et al.* 2014), musical memory is often retained (Jacobsen *et al.* 2015).

The 'deficit' framing of dementia inherent in the biomedical model is implicated in the labelling of people living with the condition as 'sufferers' and in their stigmatisation. Goffman (1963 p.3) observed that a stigmatised individual is 'reduced...from a whole and usual person to a tainted, discounted one', i.e. incapable or 'demented' and thus 'less than human'. Despite public education, a range of media often use emotionally charged and pervasive metaphors about the condition that continue to fuel a narrative of catastrophe (Zeilig 2014), which reinforces negative stereotypes and discrimination. Furthermore, Milne (2010) found that a diagnosis impacts on both individuals and their families and can negatively affect the quality of life of all involved. Hence, public information aimed at destigmatising the condition has to be carefully curated (Fletcher 2021) as highlighted by the continuing controversy around the value of *The Long Goodbye*, a video produced by the Alzheimer's Society (2024) about the experience of some family carers supporting loved ones living with the condition.

Intersectionality provides a lens for understanding how social, psychological and environmental factors shape individual and family caregiver experience of dementia. It challenges the biomedical model by recognising that the experiences of people living with the condition are also contingent on their social identities such as race, gender, class, age and disability, which intersect and influence experiences of oppression and privilege (Crenshaw 1989, 1991).

The barriers to people with memory problems from BAME communities accessing diagnosis, treatment and culturally appropriate information and support are reinforced by intersectional oppressions (Truswell 2019). Similarly, intersecting marginalised identities are implicated in negative experiences of other communities. This includes LGBTQ+ people living with dementia and their carers (Whitman and Truswell 2023), who are reluctant to approach formal services for support often because of their concerns about disclosing their identities, cognitive impairment compromising memory of sexual identity (Di Lorito *et al.* 2022). In Chapter 11 of this handbook, Allegranti (2024) highlights the importance of paying attention to the deep embeddedness of intersecting identities in ourselves and our own practice.

Psychologists use cognitive, behavioural and humanistic approaches to support individuals to maintain cognitive functioning, memory, language and orientation. They help manage behaviours associated with non-cognitive symptoms of dementia, such as depression, apathy, disinhibition and sleep disturbance. These behavioural and psychological symptoms of dementia (BPSD) are stressful for individuals and challenging for caregivers (Javed and Kakul 2023). Behavioural programmes (James and Jackson 2017) and psychosocial interventions, many of them therapies that can be helpful for people living with mild to moderate dementia, include cognitive stimulation therapy (CST) and creative arts therapies (Guss *et al.* 2014). Individualised education and support programmes for carers are effective (Cooper *et al.* 2024).

Kitwood (1997) was critical of what he called 'the standard paradigm' (*ibid.* p.1), a term that refers to the medicalisation of Alzheimer's disease with its pervasive and pessimistic view of the condition; this excludes the person – only the dementia is seen. His alternative proposition was a biopsychosocial model involving an 'interplay' between neurological impairment and psychosocial factors including health, individual psychology and the environment, with particular emphasis on social context. Using this complex, dynamic and heterogeneous notion of dementia, Kitwood and Bredin (1992) developed theories of person-centred care and personhood that changed the culture of dementia care and became the basis of best practice that underpins creative arts practice, the focus of Chapter 2.

There has been a paradigm shift in dementia care from the biomedical to a social model of disability (Fazio *et al.* 2018). The social model takes into account how social environments support or restrict the active participation of people living with dementia in society (Hare 2022). Broadening the ideas underpinning this model, Bartlett and O'Connor (2010) developed the concept of social citizenship. Social citizenship acknowledges the agency and autonomy of people living with dementia and upholds their political, civil and social rights, including the right to arts (EUAFR 2017). Importantly, Cahill (2023 p.142) asserts '[i]t is ...by framing dementia as a disability and a human rights issue, practitioners can help to change practice, inform policy and create a fairer, inclusive and more humanitarian society for all'. Practitioners and people with lived experience of dementia speaking out are in the vanguard of collective actions to drive social change in the wider socio-political sphere, including campaigning organisations such as the Scottish Dementia Working Group (SDWG) and Dementia Diarists.

The biomedical model has shaped the pharmacological research agenda, prioritising investment in medical and neuroscientific research in the search for a potential cure or disease-modifying treatment. In doing so, it has increased scientific knowledge about the human brain and behaviour. However, UK governments have shifted policy and practice to increasingly pay attention to living well with dementia. This has made psychosocial and non-pharmacological support available to meet behavioural, psychological and occupational needs in dementia and to provide effective community-based support for individuals and family carers and address barriers to access.

Research and policy around dementia prevention has accelerated. Global studies report that clinical features of the condition are affected by many other factors across the life course. Addressing 14 modifiable risk factors, which include social isolation and depression, throughout life would prevent or delay 45% of dementias diagnosed (Livingston *et al.* 2024).

The development of the field of practice

What are generally referred to as 'the arts' in the Western world have changed and evolved over decades, along with discourse about their value, function, impact and, crucially for our purposes, 'effects on people' (Belfiore and Bennett 2010 p.35). Besides being a huge source of intrinsic enjoyment and human enrichment, they have also been increasingly used instrumentally by UK governments to deliver creative services exports, many emanating from arts culture and heritage, as part of national economic plans (McAndrew *et al.* 2024). Successive administrations have supported the work of creative and cultural industries that 'have their origin in individual creativity, skill and talent and which have a potential for wealth and job creation through the generation and exploitation of intellectual property' as defined by the Department for Culture, Media and Sport, including a range of commercial occupations such as publishing and filming but also including museums, galleries and libraries (Evennett 2024).

Arts for health have been a major part of arts in life (and death) in many civilisations throughout the centuries, with art, music, dance, storytelling and drama accompanying socio-cultural rituals and used for healing. Fancourt (2017) also shows how modern developments in health and medicine promoted and supported the shift from a wholly biomedical model of health to a biopsychosocial model. This model provided opportunities for using arts to help remediate particular health conditions, enhance wellbeing, encourage healthy behaviours and address social determinants of ill health, including social isolation.

An important driver for the development of arts in health is its potential to support community health. At the local level, the community arts movement in England highlighted the social value of the arts for community development (Matarasso 1997). Arts, culture, heritage and nature have been harnessed by the government as part of place-based health initiatives that aim to prevent ill health, improve population health and wellbeing and reduce health inequalities. Early indications suggest that place-based programmes are facilitating collaborative working between public health and the arts and cultural sector (APPG AHW 2017, Fancourt and Finn 2019).

The promotion of health humanities (Coats 2004) and better evidence of the effectiveness of using arts in healthcare have contributed to its widespread adoption across multiple disciplines, including medicine, nursing, psychology and occupational therapy, and more generally by public health and a constellation of arts, culture, health and social care organisations in the statutory and Voluntary, Community and Social Enterprise (VCSE) sectors, and commercial sectors now run arts-for-health programmes for a range of conditions across the age span (APPG AHW 2017).

Over time, UK government healthcare policies have been shifting more resources from acute medical care to primary and community care, management of long-term chronic conditions and public health policies (Parkin and Baker 2021). Prevention is a priority, particularly for addressing the social determinants of health via public health education, integration of health and social care, and personalisation of care and through programmes such as social prescribing of the arts (see Chapter 13).

Arts for health progressively became aligned to these goals and policies, achieving a major milestone in the development of creative arts for health with the publication of *Creative Health: The Arts for Health and Wellbeing* produced by the All-Party Parliamentary Group on Arts, Health and Wellbeing (APPG AHW 2017). The APPG AHW (2015–2017) brought together extensive literature with the testimonial evidence of researchers, professionals, practitioners and the public about the benefits of arts for health and wellbeing for individuals, groups, communities and wider society. The implementation of the report's recommendations is now led by the National Centre for Creative Health (NCCH), a strategic organisation that seeks to embed creative health in all aspects of health commissioning and provision as an integral part of a 21st-century health and social care system. In *Creative Health Review: How*

Policy Can Embrace Creative Health (NCCH and APPG AHW 2023 p.20), creative health is defined as:

> creative approaches and activities which have benefits for our health and wellbeing… [c]reative health can contribute to the prevention of ill health, promotion of healthy behaviours, management of long-term conditions, and treatment and recovery across the life course.

To achieve this goal, the NCCH is collaborating with national arts councils, the National Academy for Social Prescribing (NASP) and the Baring Foundation and working with government departments, the NHS and social care bodies and health and social care systems including Integrated Care Boards on mechanisms and models for creative health commissioning and funding, Creative Health Practitioner workforce development (see Chapter 14) and support for Creative Health Practitioners (see Chapter 15). There is a need to address silos between Creative Practitioners and Creative Arts Therapists to improve the efficiency and effectiveness of these two key workforce groups (see Chapter 18). NCCH is partnered by the Culture, Health and Wellbeing Alliance (CHWA), a membership organisation for creative health in England. CHWA has around 6000 members and estimates that at least 10,000 people work in the field, many of them solo practitioners with people of all ages living with diverse chronic conditions in a range of settings.

Creative arts for dementia are located within the ambit of creative health. Using creative arts as a means to promote positive change in people directly affected by dementia has several roots, a number of which have already been touched on including: transformative ideas that changed the culture of care and care practice (Kitwood 1997), perception of dementia as a social disability, the human rights of people living with the condition and the campaigning work of people living with dementia. The *Journal of Dementia Care*, now Dementia Community, has championed the creative arts (Benson and Pasiecznik Parsons 2024), as have pioneers such as the poet John Killick, Julian West, who leads Music for Life at Wigmore Hall, and Susan Langford, MBE, director of Magic Me. Better evidence of the effects and benefits of the arts (Zeilig, Killick and Fox 2014, Schneider 2018), particularly music (Devere 2017), was instrumental in creative arts being recommended as a primary resource for dementia by the National Institute for Health and Care Excellence (NICE) (2018, 2019).

Creativity and dementia

Creativity and dementia are rarely linked (Brotherhood *et al.* 2017). Nevertheless, the Four C model developed by Beghetto and Kaufman (2007) offers a more nuanced view beyond the big C of 'creative genius', whose cognitive prowess results in a novel and useful product or a work of art (Csikszentmihalyi 2013). Creativity in dementia can be understood as a creative spark or mini 'c' – novel but personally meaningful creative processes, experiences and learning activities. This spark was observed in the remarkable way that care home residents with moderate cognitive impairment engaged with arts via modern technology. Working with Bo Chapman and Zoe Flynn of Frames of Mind, a small group created digital self-portraits on iPads using the Procreate app and stop-go animation to tell stories about personally meaningful material objects (Flynn and Chapman 2022), highlighting capacity for new learning. A related concept is little 'c' creativity, a growing area of research that encompasses self-expression, adaptation, day-to-day problem solving or everyday creativity (Bellas *et al.* 2019), more recently framed as leisure, i.e. 'the ways in which participation in it [daily life] enables people living with dementia to sustain their place in the world' (Gray, Russell and Twigg 2023 p.3).

Different types of dementia affect creative expression in different ways. Depending on the location of damage to the brain, it is possible that 'a unique artistic signature exists for each type of dementia diagnosis and different expressions of creativity in visual arts' (Camic *et al.* 2018 p.4). Other studies suggest that brain mechanisms and cognitive processes involved in creative arts are not irreparably damaged, emotional responses are preserved and whilst explicit memory (the ability to learn or recall events) is compromised, implicit memory (connected to emotions and feelings) is not completely lost (Savazzi *et al.* 2020).

Zeisel (2010) recognised that creative arts can help retrieve sense memories, emotional and embodied memories, hardwired memories and more that he lists in his schema called 'Memories Still There' (*ibid.* pp.11–14). Zeisel observes 'As with Marcel Proust whose memories were awakened by the taste of a madeleine at his grandmother's house – tastes, smells and visual images that can enhance access to memories of people living with Alzheimer's' (*ibid.* p.59). His schema provides a useful aide-mémoire for planning participatory arts sessions, along with prompts and cues for retrieving long-term memories and emotions. Given the trajectory of what is often referred to as 'a dementia', Camic *et al.* (2018 p.2) remind us '[a]s cognitive capacities decline and become less and less accessible, researchers and clinicians should not assume the potential for creative activity is eliminated'. We would also add national dementia leads, commissioners and managers to this list, mindful of the needs of people receiving end-of-life care.

Camic *et al.* (*ibid.* p.9) conclude their review of artistic creativity in dementia with the proposition that '[e]ven as artistic expression may change over the course of the dementias...and as cognitive abilities decline; there remain possibilities for artistic creativity to develop'. These 'possibilities' include 'in the moment' creative experiences – authentic but transient experiences noted by families, practitioners and researchers (MacPherson *et al.* 2009, Keady *et al.* 2022).

Making the case for differentiating objective forms of creativity (product) and subjective forms of creativity (process), Stein (1953 p.311) cautions 'against overlooking necessary distinction between the creative product and the creative experience'. In focusing on the experience rather than on making or creating (something) artistic, creativity becomes 'failure free' (Swinnen and de Medeiros 2018). The focus of all work with people living with dementia is the process, social relationships and relational interactions (Kitwood 1993, Killick and Craig 2011). Good practice involves levelling power relationships, i.e. working non-hierarchically, sharing the creative task and erasing distinctions between the producer (artist) and the participant (Zeilig, West and van der Byl Williams 2018). A more recent study focuses on the active role played by the artists who are integral to process, noting that improvisation plays a key part (West *et al.* 2023), hence the need for facilitators to foster opportunities for supporting participants to take on co-created leadership/facilitation roles and being mindful that 'individuals with dementia can make recognisably creative contributions despite the absence of sensical language' (Kontos, Miller and Kontos 2017 p.188).

Defining creative arts practice

Ultimately, creativity in the arts offers a medium for enabling people with cognitive impairment to connect with and express their emotions, feelings and experiences in a way that is not dependent on memory, prior skill or even interest (Basting 2009). Indeed, Hayes (2011) describes creativity as an essential energy, for it comes:

> ...from somewhere beyond the intellect; it flows from an intuitive non-rational place in the body and mind and we [as practitioners] can tap into the creativity of everyone, no matter how much their logic or sequential memory has been disturbed. (p.15)

This is reflected in our working definition of creative arts practice:

> The purposeful application of person-centred values to creative arts practice which engages with, and relates to, people living with dementia in ways that facilitate meaningful, imaginative, and emotional experience and promote

health and wellbeing. Creative arts include both direct participation and/or non-direct appreciative involvement in cultural, heritage and nature activities and experiences.

The range of artistic disciplines involved include painting, drawing and crafting, digital arts and music including singing, playing and listening, dance and movement, creative writing especially poetry, storytelling and reminiscence using prompts such as music, objects, and sensory stimuli. The diversity and richness of what arts and culture can offer for people living with the condition includes facilitating the body's interaction with the artistic stimulus. Whether in the fine motor skills required in marquetry, basketry and music making, or the fine and gross motor skills in movement and dance, the importance of the body and non-verbal communications cannot be underestimated when verbal communication and cognitive skills are compromised. Hence:

> The goal of the creative-expressive approach is to reach beyond the confusion, conveying love, respect and understanding while celebrating the fragments of thought, memory feeling and movement that arise. When we do this, we also touch the deeper parts of our own selves. (Coaten 2001 p.22)

Indirect (appreciative) participation takes place in arts and cultural venues, many of which have become dementia friendly (Allen *et al.* 2015), where museum collections, exhibitions, plays and heritage arts are accessed in ways that support the involvement of participants with different needs, abilities and strengths, with positive results for wellbeing (Camic, Tischler and Pearman 2014). Increasingly, arts organisations offer nature-based experiences, such as the walks organised by the Sensory Trust in Cornwall and Alive Activities in Bristol, who run a multisensory allotment project.

Practitioners, backgrounds and settings

We use Creative Health Practitioners (CHPs) as a collective term to refer to two specific groups of practitioners and facilitators: Creative Arts Therapists (CATs) and Creative Practitioners (CPs). Whilst acknowledging the distinctiveness of CATs, we are inclined to agree with Fancourt and Finn (2019), who include arts therapies within creative health care, as they are used as a medium for supporting individuals' health and wellbeing. We are aware of the need to optimise available resources, and in Chapter 18, we call for more creative dialogue between these practitioners.

CATs hold postgraduate qualifications and are professionally registered art, music or drama therapists or Dance Movement Psychotherapists (DMPs) who work mainly in healthcare and education settings and receive clinical supervision. Increasing numbers work in community settings, often as free-lancers (see Chapter 17).

CPs are often trained in an art form but have a wide range of backgrounds and qualifications. They usually learn by experience whilst working in the community for arts, music and dance centres, charities and cultural venues and in day centres, care homes, hospitals and hospices. Most do not have for-mal support and supervision provided by employers. A number of CPs work as activity coordinators, healthcare assistants and outreach leads for cultural venues. Chapter 14 examines the creative health workforce, and Chapter 15 explores self-care and support.

How the creative health practice is funded

A number of (large, national) arts and culture infrastructure organisations and providers are National Portfolio Organisations. These receive pub-lic (government) funding awarded by national arts councils. The majority (mainly small, medium and micro-organisations, including many charities) are reliant on securing several sources of funding. Funding comes from national arts councils, charitable trusts, local community foundations and businesses or through corporate giving, donations and events. Local councils are the biggest public funder of arts and culture, but the overall decline in local government revenue expenditure has significantly impacted on support for arts and culture projects and programmes. With it, employment oppor-tunities for CHPs have reduced.

Since the 1970s, global socio-economic crises have increasingly impacted on public funding of arts and culture provision resulting in government and cultural sector policies shifting to helping national and local organisations diversify income and build new revenue streams to mitigate funding short-falls. For example, in setting out its investment principles, Arts Council Eng-land (ACE) stated that cultural organisations will 'develop business models that help them maximise income, reduce costs and become more financially resilient' (ACE 2020 p.49).

Conclusion

The artist Matisse is credited with saying 'Creativity takes courage.' This returns us to Keith Oliver's profound words. These words go to the heart of what we must do as CHPs if we are to connect with Keith and with many thousands of other individuals in ways that help to facilitate living a creative life to the full.

We set out to contextualise creative arts and dementia, creative arts for dementia and creative arts in dementia. We began with an overview of the dialectics of dementia, summarising the biomedical model. We noted the critiques drawn from psychological, social, environmental and intersectional perspectives, which concluded with support for a biopsychosocial model. The focus then shifted to the development of the arts for health and its drivers, many of which chime with the growth of creative arts in dementia. We noted the multiple drivers for the development of creative arts in engaging with people living with dementia, defined creative arts practice, listed the creative arts and described CHPs who make up the workforce, where they work and how they are funded. Both organisations and CHPs continue to be affected by cuts in public funding, and that funding remains a major concern. However, overall, there is a strong case for locating this work in the ambit of creative health.

Dementia is a major public health issue in the UK and worldwide. Many of the needs of people living with dementia and their family carers can be met in part through taking part in creative arts. Although creative arts are not curative, there is much that they can offer on a day which, post diagnosis, may be devoid of meaningful occupation and social connections. This chapter has shown how creativity brings arts to life whilst those that follow describe, more fully, the benefits for health and wellbeing.

LEARNING POINTS

We, as practitioners, managers, commissioners and others, need to listen to people living with the condition and enable them to live the lives they want to live. This chapter scaffolds the rest of the handbook in that:

- CPs require an understanding of the biopsychosocial model of dementia.

- It is important to take into account dementia, which impacts on a person's identity and exacerbates other intersectional aspects such as race, gender, class, culture and stigma.

- In the absence of a cure or effective disease-modifying treatment, creative arts offer opportunities to maintain quality of life, health and wellbeing, and staying active and involved in the community.

References

Allegranti, B. (2024) *Moving Kinship: Practicing Feminist Justice in a More-than-Human World.* London: Routledge.

Allen, P., Brown, A., Camic, P. M., Cutler, D., *et al.* (2015) *Dementia Friendly Arts Guide: A Practical Guide to Becoming A Dementia-Friendly Arts Venue.* London: Alzheimer's Society.

Alzheimer's Research UK (2024) Dementia statistics hub. https://dementiastatistics.org/about-dementia/prevalence-and-incidence

Alzheimer's Society (2024) The Long Goodbye: our new advert. www.alzheimers.org.uk/about-us/dementia-news-and-media/long-goodbye

Alzheimer's Society (2025) Dementia medication. www.alzheimers.org.uk/about-dementia/treatments/dementia-medication

Alzheimer's Society and Carnall Farrar (2024) *The Economic Impact of Dementia.* Alzheimer's Society: London. www.carnallfarrar.com/wp-content/uploads/2024/06/The-economic-impact-of-dementia-CF.pdf

APPG AHW (All-Party Parliamentary Group on Arts, Health and Wellbeing) (2017) *Creative Health: The Arts for Health and Wellbeing.* 2nd edition. www.artshealthandwellbeing.org.uk/appg-inquiry

APPG Dementia (All-Party Parliamentary Group on Dementia) (2013) *Dementia Does Not Discriminate: The Experience of Black, Asian and Minority Ethnic Communities.* London: Alzheimer's Society.

Bartlett, R. and O'Connor, D. (2010) *Broadening the Dementia Debate.* Bristol: Bristol University Press.

Basting, A. (2009) *Forget Memory: Creating Better Lives for People with Dementia.* Baltimore, MD: John Hopkins University Press.

Beghetto, R. A. and Kaufman, J. C. (2007) 'Toward a broader conception of creativity: A case for "mini-c" creativity.' *Psychology of Aesthetics, Creativity, and the Arts* 1, 2, 73–79.

Belfiore, E. and Bennett, O. (2010) *The Social Impact of the Arts.* Basingstoke: Palgrave Macmillan.

Bellass, S., Balmer, A., May, V., Keady, J. *et al.* (2019) 'Broadening the debate on creativity and dementia: A critical approach.' *Dementia* 18, 7–8, 2799–2820.

Benson, S. and Pasiecznik Parsons, M. (2024) 'A celebration of the arts.' *Journal of Dementia Care*, November/December, special issue. https://journalofdementiacare.co.uk/issue/november-december-2024

Bond, J. (2001) 'Sociological Perspectives.' In C. Cantley (2001) (ed.) *A Handbook of Dementia Care.* Buckingham: Open University Press.

Brotherhood, E., Ball, P., Camic, P. M., Evans, C. *et al.* (2017) 'Preparatory planning framework for Created Out of Mind.' *Wellcome Open Research.* DOI: 10.12688/wellcomeopenres.12773.1

Cahill, S. (2023) 'Dementia and Human Rights.' In M. Krennerich, M. Lissowsky and M. Schendel (2023) (eds) *Die Freiheit der Menschenrechte. Wochen Schau Wissenschaft.* Wochen Schau Wissenschaft.

Camic, P., Tischler, V. and Pearman, C. (2013) 'Viewing and making art together: A multi-session art-gallery-based intervention for people with dementia and their carers.' *Aging Mental Health* 18, 2, 161–168.

Camic, P. M., Crutch, S. J., Murphy, C., Firth, N. C. *et al.* (Created Out of Mind Team) (2018) 'Conceptualising and understanding artistic creativity in the dementias: Interdisciplinary approaches to research and practise.' *Frontiers Psychology* 3, 9, 1842.

Carter, J. (2022) 'Prevalence of all cause young onset dementia and time lived with dementia: Analysis of primary care.' *Journal of Dementia Care* 30, 3, 1–5.

Coaten, R. (2001) 'Exploring reminiscence through dance and movement.' *Journal of Dementia Care* 9, 5 19–22.

Coats, E. (2004) *Creative Arts and Humanities in Healthcare: Swallows to Other Continents.* London: The Nuffield Trust.

Cooper, C., Vickerstaff, V., Barber, J., Phillips, R. *et al.* (2024) 'A psychosocial goal-setting and manualised support intervention for independence in dementia (NIDUS-Family) versus goal setting and routine care: A single-masked, phase 3, superiority, randomised controlled trial.' *The Lancet Healthy Longevity* 5, 2, 141–151.

Crenshaw, K. (1989) 'Demarginalizing the intersection of race and sex: A Black feminist critique of antidiscrimination doctrine, feminist theory and antiracist politics.' *University
of Chicago Legal Forum,* 139, 139–168.

Crenshaw, K. (1991) 'Mapping the margins: Intersectionality, identity politics, and violence
against women of color.' *Stanford Law Review* 43, 6, 1241–1299.

Csikszentmihalyi, M. (2013) *Creativity: The Psychology of Discovery and Invention.* New
York: Harper Perennial Modern Classics.

Dementia UK (2025) Young onset dementia. www.dementiauk.org/information-and-support/
young-onset-dementia

Devere, R. (2017) 'Music and dementia: An overview.' *Practical Neurology.* https://practical-
neurology.com/articles/2017-june/music-and-dementia-an-overview

Di Lorito, C., Bosco, A., Peel, E., Hinchliff, S., *et al.* (2022) 'Are dementia services and support
organisations meeting the needs of Lesbian, Gay, Bisexual and Transgender (LGBT) caregivers of LGBT people living with dementia? A scoping review of the literature.' *Aging
& Mental Health* 26, 10, 1912–1921.

EUAFR (European Union Agency for Fundamental Rights) (2017) *Exploring the Connections
Between Arts and Human Rights: Report of High-Level Expert Meeting, Vienna, 29–30 May
2017.* https://fra.europa.eu/sites/default/files/fra_uploads/fra-2017_arts-and-human-rights-
report_may-2017_vienna.pdf

Evennett, H. (2024) In focus: contribution of the arts to society and the economy. https://
lordslibrary.parliament.uk/contribution-of-the-arts-to-society-and-the-economy

Fancourt, D. (2017) *Arts in Health: Designing and Researching Interventions.* Oxford: Oxford
University Press.

Fancourt, D. and Finn, S. (2019) *What Is the Evidence on the Role of the Arts in Improving Health
and Well-Being? A Scoping Review.* Health Evidence Network (HEN) Synthesis Report 67.
Copenhagen: WHO Regional Office for Europe.

Fazio, S., Pace, D., Flinner, J. and Kallmyer, B. (2018) 'The fundamentals of person-centered
care for individuals with dementia.' *Gerontologist* 18, 58 (suppl 1), S10–S19.

Fletcher, J. R. (2021) 'Destigmatising dementia: The dangers of felt stigma and benevolent
othering.' *Dementia* 20, 2, 417–426.

Flynn, Z. and Chapman, B. (2022) 'Frames of Mind: Bringing Memories to Life with Stop Go
Animation.' In I. Parker, R. Coaten and M. Hopfenbeck (eds) *The Practical Handbook of
Living with Dementia.* Monmouth: PCCS Books.

Giebel, C., Sutcliffe, C., Stolt, M. and Karlsson, S. *et al.* (2014) 'Deterioration of basic activities of daily living and their impact on quality of life across different cognitive stages of
dementia: A European study.' *International Psychogeriatrics* 26, 8, 1283–1293.

Goffman, E. (1963) *Stigma Notes on the Management of Spoiled Identity.* London: Penguin.

Gray, K., Russell, C. and Twigg, J. (2024) *Leisure and Everyday Life with Dementia.* Maiden-
head: Open University Press.

Guss, R. with Alzheimer's Society, Dementia Action Alliance, Dementia Engagement and
Empowerment Project (DEEP) and people living with dementia and the Dementia Work
Stream Expert Reference Group (2014) *A Guide to Psychosocial Interventions in Early Stages
of Dementia.* Leicester: British Society of Psychology Division of Clinical Psychology Fac-
ulty of the Psychology of Older People.

Hare, P. (2022) *Dementia, Disability and Hope: How Can We Embed Change Together?* Innovations in Dementia. www.innovationsindementia.org.uk/wp-content/uploads/2022/02/
Dementia-Disability-and-Hope-2.pdf

Hayes, J. with Povey, S. (2011) *The Creative Arts in Dementia Care.* London: Jessica Kingsley
Publishers.

Jacobsen, J. H, Stelzer, J., Fritz, T. H., Chételat, G., La Joie, R. and Turner, R. (2015) 'Why musical memory can be preserved in advanced Alzheimer's disease.' *Brain* 138, 8, 2438–2450.

James, I. and Jackson, L. (2017) *Understanding Behaviour in Dementia that Challenges.* 2nd
edition. London: Jessica Kingsley Publishers.

Javed, S. and Kakul, F. (2023) 'Psychological theories of dementia.' *Journal of Gerontology and
Geriatrics* 17, 2, 104–114.

Journal of Dementia Care (2024) NHS England include dementia in their 2024/25 objectives. https://journalofdementiacare.co.uk/nhs-england-objectives

Keady, J. D., Campbell, S., Clark, A., Dowlen, R. *et al.* (2022) 'Re-thinking and re-positioning "being in the moment" within a continuum of moments: Introducing a new conceptual framework for dementia studies.' *Ageing and Society, 42,* 3, 681–702.

Killick, J. and Craig, C. (2011) *Creativity and Communication in Persons with Dementia: A Practical Guide.* London: Jessica Kingsley Press.

Kitwood, T. (1993) 'Person and process in dementia.' *International Journal of Geriatric Psychiatry 8,* 7, 541–545.

Kitwood, T. (1997) *Dementia Reconsidered: The Person Comes First.* Buckingham: Open University Press.

Kitwood, T. and Bredin, K. (eds) (1992) 'Towards a theory of dementia care personhood and well-being.' *Ageing and Society 12,* 269–287.

Kontos, P., Miller, K.-L. and Kontos, A. (2017) 'Relational citizenship: Supporting embodied selfhood and relationality in dementia care.' *Sociology of Health Illness 39,* 2, 182–198.

Livingston, G., Huntley, J., Lui, Y., Costafreda, S. G., *et al.* (2024) 'Dementia prevention, intervention, and care: 2024 report of the Lancet standing commission.' *The Lancet 404,* 10452, 572–628.

Long, S., Benoist, C. and Weidner, W. (2023) *World Alzheimer Report. Reducing Dementia Risk: Never Too Early, Never Too Late.* London: Alzheimer's Disease International. www.alzint.org/u/World-Alzheimer-Report-2023.pdf

MacPherson, S., Bird, M., Anderson, K., Davis, T. and Blair, A. (2009) 'An art gallery access programme for people with dementia: "You do it for the moment".' *Ageing Mental Health 13,* 744–752.

McAndrew, S., O'Brien, D., Taylor, M. and Wang, R. (2024) *Arts, Culture and Heritage: Audiences and Workforce.* Newcastle: Creative Industries Policy and Evidence Centre. https://pec.ac.uk/state_of_the_nation/arts-cultural-heritage-audiences-and-workforce-2

Manthorpe, J. and Iliffe, S. (2016) *The Dialectics of Dementia.* London: King's College London.

Matarasso, F. (1997) *Use or Ornament? The Social Impact of Participation in the Arts.* Stroud: Comedia.

Milne, A. (2010) 'The "D" word: Reflections on the relationship between stigma, discrimination and dementia.' *Journal of Mental Health 19,* 3, 227–233.

Mukadam, N., Marston, L., Lewis, G. and Livingston, G. (2022) 'Risk factors, ethnicity and dementia: A UK Biobank prospective cohort study of White, South Asian and Black participants.' *PLOS ONE 17,* 10.

National Institute for Health and Care Excellence (2018) *Dementia: Assessment, Management and Support for People Living with Dementia and Their Carers.* NICE Guidance (NG97). www.nice.org.uk/guidance/ng97

National Institute for Health and Care Excellence (2019) *Dementia. Quality Standard* (QS184). www.nice.org.uk/guidance/qs184/chapter/quality-statement-5-activities-to-promote-wellbeing#quality-statement-5-activities-to-promote-wellbeing

National Institute for Health and Care Excellence (2025) Dementia: how common is it? https://cks.nice.org.uk/topics/dementia/background-information/prevalence

NCCH and APPG AHW (National Centre for Creative Health and the All-Party Parliamentary Group on Arts, Health, and Wellbeing) (2023) *Creative Health Review: How Policy Can Embrace Creative Health.* https://ncch.org.uk/creative-health-review

Oliver, K. (2019) *Dear Alzheimer's: A Diary of Living with Dementia.* London: Jessica Kingsley Publishers.

Oung, C., Lobont, C. and Curry, N. (2024) *What Needs to Improve for Social Care to Better Support People with Dementia?* London: The Nuffield Trust. www.nuffieldtrust.org.uk/research/what-needs-to-improve-for-social-care-to-better-support-people-with-dementia

Parkin, E. and Baker, C. (2021) *Dementia Policy Care and Statistics.* House of Commons Library Briefing Paper 70007, 14 May.

Stein, M. I. (1953) 'Creativity and culture.' *Journal of Psychology 36,* 311–322.

Swinnen, A. and de Medeiros, K. (2018) '"Play" and people living with dementia: A humanities-based inquiry of timeslips and the Alzheimer's Poetry Project.' *Gerontologist 58,* 2, 261–269.

Truswell, D. (ed.) (2019) *Supporting People Living with Dementia in Black, Asian and Minority Ethnic Communities: Key Issues and Strategies for Change.* London: Jessica Kingsley Publishers.

West, J., Zeilig, H., Cape, T. and Payne, L. (2023) 'Making a living moment more resonant: An exploration of the role of the artist in co-creative work with people living with dementia.' *Wellcome Open Research.* https://wellcomeopenresearch.org/articles/8-580

Whitman, L. and Truswell, D. (2023) 'Equality, diversity and inclusion: A special issue.' *Journal of Dementia Care 31*, 5. https://journalofdementiacare.co.uk/wp-content/uploads/2023/10/JDCSEPT23.pdf

Zeilig, H. (2014) 'Dementia as a cultural metaphor.' *Gerontologist 54*, 2, 258–267.

Zeilig, H., West, J. and van der Byl Williams, M. (2018) 'Co-creativity: possibilities for using the arts with people with a dementia.' *Quality in Ageing and Older Adults 19*, 2, 135–145.

Zeisel, J. (2010) *I'm Still Here: A Breakthrough Approach to Understanding Someone Living with Alzheimer's.* London: Piatkus, Little Brown Book Group.

CHAPTER 2

Reflecting on Good Practice in Creative Arts and Dementia

Richard Coaten and Maria Pasiecznik Parsons

Introduction

What do guidelines for good practice look and feel like? Whether someone is just starting out or highly experienced, is there something here that inspires interest, confidence and, hopefully, curiosity? We are talking about bringing wide-ranging art forms, practitioners and skill sets to the table, from creative arts therapies through to Creative Practitioners (CPs), in many different settings. It's challenging, and this is a handbook not a manual, so its purpose must be to focus on what is most important to know in the context of Chapter 1 and what is to follow.

We begin with that powerful maxim that should be ringing in all our ears: 'Nothing About Us Without Us' (Charlton 1998). The title of what is arguably the first book in the literature on disability oppression and empowerment is now in common usage with people living with the condition and their carers. A powerful remembrance for all of us in the field for two reasons and as a foundation for what follows:

- If the psychology of relationships is left out of the equation in trying to understand dementia syndrome better, then there is no place for the context and environment, including the social and psychological within which the condition plays out. There is no place, in other words, for giving people with dementia a sense that, in spite of their condition, there is much that can still be accomplished – creatively, socially, psychologically, culturally and environmentally, enabling them to cope better. Our starting point must be to continue to use as many of the individual resources that remain relatively unaffected and to put the person with dementia in control, living a life that is as full and rich as possible. Within this psychosocial paradigm there remains the presence of *hope* – the ongoing possibility that they are still human beings, still making sense of their world as best they can and still having the wherewithal to banish the shame, fear and isolation, particularly in how it is perceived in society. It is within this frame that all our creative work finds a culture, a home and values that understand and encourage its development (see next paragraph).

- Michael Verde (cited in Greenblat 2011) from Memory Bridge (USA) speaks powerfully to how people in society generally view the condition and the need to learn how to banish the shame, fear and isolation. He argues that in everyday communications, our egos are habituated to this maxim: 'I'll reflect you back to you, if you reflect me back to me' (p.88). However, the subtleties in this process become harder and harder for people with cognitive losses, and when they reach this stage, are described as having 'gone' (p.88). He maintains that if we want to make the 'gone' reappear, then, without a cure, we have to get our own egos out of the way. Here is how to do it:

    The next time you communicate with someone who is not at his or her cognitive best, remind yourself of this:

    This interaction is not about me. This interaction is about someone who is seeking connections on terms that may not advance the interests or needs of my ego. I am going to go where your needs are taking you. I am going to be with you in that place, wherever and however it is. I am going to let my ego disappear now. I am going to love you in your image instead of trying to re-create you in mine. (p.88)

Based on these two credos, this chapter shines a light on good practice in using creative arts informed by person-centredness (Kitwood and Bredin 1992). Whilst person-centredness is the cornerstone of good practice in creative arts and dementia, we also highlight the importance of working to clear standards and values that inform it. This work also involves family carers, their friends and professional care staff. Empowering carers to be creative is an important component of good practice, and gives them knowledge and skills that may support their resilience, coping and improvisational strategies (Coaten 2022, cited in Parker, Coaten and Hopfenbeck 2022).

This chapter cannot cover the whole large field; instead, it draws the reader's attention to the 'How' concerning core values, skills and knowledge that underpin all that we do, since if you have the 'How' firmly rooted, then the 'What' will take care of itself.

Definitions

'Best practice' is an approach or a method that has been generally accepted as preferable to known alternatives, because it usually produces results superior to those achieved by other means or because it has become a standard way of doing things. When this practice becomes established (used by the group for which it was recommended), it becomes a good practice, the implication being that it is automatically followed by everyone concerned. For example, the National Institute for Health and Care Excellence (NICE) produces standards for the NHS that are explicit as to whether a treatment or intervention should be 'offered', based on clear and strong evidence, or whether it should be 'considered' when the evidence is less strong. (See NICE's Dementia Quality Standard (2019) and also Chapters 1 and 18.)

This chapter speaks to both Creative Arts Therapists (CATs) and CPs working in the field and proposes a great deal more collaboration and dialogue, discussed further in Chapter 18. However, many arts therapists, including Richard, started out as practising artists, moving on to become therapists later. Importantly, this does not prevent them from working as either CPs or CATs, circumstances depending. Now, we look at a philosophical and practical home and set of values for our work, whether we practise as a CAT, a CP or a combination of the two.

Locating a culture, a home and values for our work in person-centred care

Person-centred care (PCC) has its origins in the work of Carl Rogers, whose person-centred counselling approach emphasises the importance of a counsellor's 'unconditional positive regard' for the person and viewing them holistically (Rogers 2004). Professor Tom Kitwood and colleagues at the Bradford Dementia Group in the 1990s built on these roots. They stressed the importance of seeing *the person first*: by shifting our gaze from the person with *dementia* to the *person* with dementia. Kitwood developed several explanatory concepts, including a vital set of values, emphasising that the *person's* interests are at the heart of every interaction and caring act.

The concept of personhood is central to PCC. It is defined as '[a] standing or status that is bestowed upon one human being by others, in the context of relationship and social being. It implies recognition, respect and trust'

(Kitwood 1997 p.8). Kitwood points to 'our common ground' (1997 p.6), asking readers 'to take a long hard look at what and who someone with dementia was, and still is, in terms of humanity. He [Kitwood] wanted to show that "they" are "us" and "we" are "them" and any contrived separation was artificial' (Dewing 2019 p.18).

Kitwood used a visual metaphor, to express his '...five great needs which overlap, coming together in the central need for love...' (1997 p.81) (see Figure 2.1). This theme is also echoed by Verde. Here, each petal represents a different need for maintaining personhood, and they operate like a 'co-operative' (*ibid.* p.81):

- Love – unconditional acceptance and empathy.
- Comfort – the feeling of trust that comes from others.
- Attachment – security and finding familiarity in unusual places.
- Inclusion – being involved in the lives of others.
- Occupation – being involved in the processes of normal life.
- Identity – that distinguishes a person from others and makes them unique.

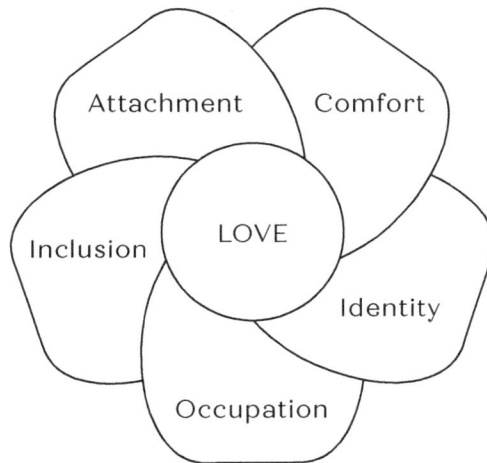

Figure 2.1 *The needs of people living with dementia*
REPRODUCED USING THE DRAWING IN KITWOOD 1997 P.82

Kitwood's enriched model of dementia (1997) challenged the 'standard paradigm' of the biomedical model of dementia by using a *biopsychosocial* perspective. Each person has a different experience dependent on the interplay between their neurological impairment, health and physical fitness, biography/life history, personality and social psychology (social context). In using this approach, caregivers who *get to know* the person optimise their wellbeing and quality of life.

Nevertheless, caregivers might, through carelessness or fatigue, undermine personhood by interacting in ways that Kitwood (*ibid.*) called a Malignant Social Psychology (MSP). Feelings or experiences of the person are dismissed or ignored, leaving them demoralised. MSP includes behaviours such as intimidation, outpacing, treachery and disempowerment (*ibid.* p.47). To counter MSP, Kitwood (*ibid.*) proposed 'Positive Person Work'. Positive Person Work acknowledges the person as a unique individual. It provides opportunities for them to engage with and negotiate decisions about their care via 'personal enhancers' that improve wellbeing and maintain personhood. These include warmth, holding, relaxed pace and respect (*ibid.* pp.90–91).

Brooker (2007) and then Brooker and Latham (2016) developed the VIPS framework to clarify and update Kitwood's ideas. The acronym VIPS describes how people with dementia and their carers must be 'Valued', be treated as 'Individuals', have their 'Perspective' respected, and how we must also attend to their 'Social environment'.

Providing a supportive social environment is key to helping maintain personhood on a day-to-day basis during the trajectory of the condition. It recognises that all human life is grounded in relationships and an enriched social environment is crucial in fostering opportunities for personal growth, while making significant compensation for any impairments. Practitioners may find reference to the VIPS framework an important aide-mémoire for practice, especially when considering how their work also enriches the social environment and supports wellbeing.

The PCC framework provides a culture, home and profoundly important set of values for how to situate our practice. The long list of creative practices referred to in Chapter 1 makes four distinct contributions to the field.

- First, as a *vehicle* for the self to be enabled to engage creatively in life-affirming ways through all the art forms.
- Second, as a vitally important *relational bridge* between people living with the condition and their caregivers, where each can see and value the other in ways that facilitate connection, relationship and creative expression.
- Third, in *healing* by helping remake a sense of the whole (person) through connecting the self with caregivers (Hayes 2011, Innes and Hatfield 2002).
- Fourth, by way of the importance of what we call embodied practices

(Coaten 2009), or what Kontos (2006) has called 'embodied selfhood', those that centre on relational and affective non-verbal communications where cognition is impaired (see Chapter 5 and Chapter 11).

For the practitioner working in a person-centred way, it means applying co-production and co-creation and 'Nothing About Us Without Us' (Charlton 1998) throughout. Sessions are tailored to individual needs, to the strengths, abilities and interests of people living with the condition, and well-paced, whether working with individuals or in a group.

Standards of practice: the Creative Health Quality Framework

There have been many positive changes to the practice and policy frameworks within the arts and health field, especially since the APPG AHW *Creative Health* report (2017). A significant one is the Culture, Health and Wellbeing Alliance's Creative Health Quality Framework (CHQF) (2023), a set of principles that underlie good practice. In summary, it is a framework built from a set of key guiding principles, 'articulating what good looks like across the creative, cultural and health sectors' (p.3), created after extensive collaboration and road-testing by over 200 artists, researchers and health commissioners in the creative health sector.

Practice does not happen in a vacuum. The CHQF is a step forward in meeting the needs of policy makers, commissioners, funders, organisations and practitioners in relation to quality standards. This framework is an excellent basis for the work we describe in this chapter. It is easily accessible online. Here, we provide some examples in a more specific dementia context, including some key elements for those just starting out on this journey.

Making what we do equitable (Culture, Health and Wellbeing Alliance 2023)

Being person-centred is the first guiding principle of the framework. The second is making what we do equitable: supporting equity, social and climate justice. Awareness of what we do in relation to diversity and inclusion is also vital. This links strongly with awareness of intersectionality (see Chapters 1 and 11), which requires that practitioners take account of health inequalities, socio-economic deprivation and other factors that individuals living with the condition will be experiencing. These are three examples of the eight guiding principles and their links to practice in this field that we consider to have a particular relevance to arts-based practice in this field. Please refer to the document itself for the others.

We are now going to discuss identifying core knowledge and skills.

Identifying core knowledge and skills
Attunement
A core skill for the practitioner is to have the time, patience and trust in oneself to 'attune'. This means recognising and engaging with another's physical, emotional and psychological state. For example, being as open to non-verbal communications as one is to verbal communications, making eye contact with everyone and developing what might be called an embodied empathy, where we pay close attention to the dynamics of moving bodies in relation to space, time and effort. Richard likes to do this at the beginning of a session. Asking them their name, he invites participants, with music playing, to move or dance with him to a chair. He thus discovers their mood, the presence of any ailments, aches or pains and their level of ability to move rhythmically. He can remember their movement characteristics and whether they engaged for later, while, importantly, at the same time learning their names.

Kitwood articulates this process of attunement well, describing slowing down and having the patience to develop what he calls a 'poetic awareness':

> We need to slow down our thought processes, to become inwardly quiet, and to have a kind of poetic awareness: that is, to look for the significance of metaphor and allusion rather than pursuing meaning with a relentless kind of tunnel vision. (Kitwood 1997 p.51)

Not only does this speak to the poetic qualities of attunement and empathy, but becoming inwardly quiet is also another way of putting what Richard has described as being 'Creatively Alert' (Coaten and Warren 2008). In other words, attentive to the creative ideas, memories, conversations, movement metaphors and allusions as they emerge.

Metaphor, allusion and symbolism
John Killick, a specialist in creative writing, argues that the condition has a disinhibiting effect on the speech of many people. As a result, barriers to emotional expression are lifted. In consequence, he reports that '[s]uddenly talk blooms with metaphor, allusion, the currents of feeling are reflected in rhythm and cadence. I have no doubt that the natural language of those with dementia is poetry' (Killick 1997 p.7). Here, people's inner feelings, unconscious desires, wants and needs become expressed metaphorically or

symbolically by a poem, a movement phrase, a work of art, improvised music or theatre improvisation. This in turn gives the practitioner the ability to work in multi-modal embodied, artistic, poetic, musical and dramatic ways to enable communication of that for which there may be no other legitimate form of expression (Coaten 2009). From Richard's experience, as the condition develops, we need to attend more to the creative, improvisational, embodied, non-verbal, emotional and symbolic ways people will communicate with us and be there for them when they do so. This is a big ask but potentially immensely rewarding for all parties. This is the principal reason Richard has stayed in the field for 40 years.

Holding a creative group space

Embedded in previous paragraphs are qualities of acceptance, openness to creative possibility within a values-based framework of person-centredness and nurturing our creative selves. All are necessary when holding the space. When Richard started out, he always began with a plan, thinking that this was what he needed to 'do' to give the session a coherent structure. He already had the frame of a Warm-Up, Central Development and Closure (Chaiklin and Schmais 1986). However, he became so focused on controlling it that he didn't know how to manage what he understood at the time to be frustrating variables. Participants would come and go, watch the birds out of the window or try to work his sound device for him. He found the whole thing very stressful. He later co-wrote about the experience with a Dance Movement Psychotherapist (DMP) colleague who was just starting out years after Richard began (Coaten and Williams 2016) and who had very similar experiences.

Richard learned to prepare the session in great detail, which provided comfort or reassurance. However, once you are in the room with the group, let it all go, forget it. Be fully present in the space, in the moment. Trust your intuition and enjoy being open to what may spontaneously come from the group. It means being open to 'relationship' and the possibility of getting to know members of the group and valuing whatever it is they bring. In between the activities, there will be opportunities to reflect on proceedings and provide necessary breathing space. Richard has transformed from a practitioner needing order in structure, content and form, scared of difference and diversity, to one who now relishes what the differences, ambiguity and diversity might offer. Remember, in that unrushed open space, something new can happen, can be co-created, which quite simply might be all that remains for the person.

Vignette – a focus on the *how*

This vignette provides an example in the form of feedback from a family member about Richard's work as a DMP in a healthcare environment. Rachel, the family member, was also a CAT and a colleague, and knew from the 'inside' what was happening, its rationale and its impact. The quality of feedback like this in practice is rare. Richard remains indebted to Rachel as a colleague for the 'mirror' she held up to his practice. He also thanks her for writing and sharing about it with such clarity, as did other members of her family, and for giving permission for her words to be placed here.

Richard was able to meet Dad on a number of levels:

- Establish a respectful and somewhat deferential relationship with dad (my assumption is that he was able to work within the transference and respond to Dad's emotional and relational needs – that of the teacher and carer – not the one needing care).

- Help dad make relationships on the ward non-verbally.

- Play...within this playing, Dad was able to 'act out' some of his anger and fear and work through these tricky emotions safely.

- Help us as a family to establish and to some extent heal our very difficult and disjointed relationships with him...he was a difficult father with many faults but there was much love entwined in this difficulty. I think I engaged less than the other two in the movement therapy – partly perhaps because I was somewhat professionally connected and also as I was keeping my child/needy self more hidden as I was his carer and 'mother' figure (he often called me mom). (personal communication)

Sharing a small part of this journey shines a light on the importance of building relationships, working non-verbally, within sound ethical practices underpinned by a set of values informed by 'personhood' (Kitwood and Bredin 1992). It must also be said that people can be reached in similar ways by CATs, CPs and others using different art forms. Crucially, here, relationships also involved family members and carers. The difference the work made to this one very vulnerable older person and his family in his last days was deeply humbling. The narratives, processes and results of this work often do not have the necessary consent to be disseminated. Without them, however, it is hard for anyone outside of the CAT frame to know what these practices entail, since the outlets for these communications usually remain the preserve of respective CAT journals.

Conclusion

It was in 2000 that Kitwood described how knowledge about how to care well for people living with the condition was growing and that '[a]s each new discovery is made, it is as if we are finding the different pieces that make up a vast mosaic; and as we begin to fit them together, a beautiful, elaborate and mysterious pattern is taking shape' (Kitwood 2000 p.9). All CPs and CATs are working as members of a community of practice that can be seen as a growing and beautiful mosaic. If Kitwood is right, then each new piece we discover will be '...a source of fresh strength and confidence; [and]...will shine like a jewel in the light' (*ibid.* p.9). If as a community of practice, we bring a 'source of fresh strength and confidence' (*ibid.* p.9) to those with whom we work, and we can demonstrate clearly to ourselves and others that we are doing that, then we are helping change the culture of dementia care and reducing fear, stigma and isolation so that we all can shine like jewels in the light.

LEARNING POINTS

- At the heart of person-centredness are values that help rekindle kindness, compassion, respect for a shared humanity and inspiration through creative dialogue in an art form at the centre of which is 'relationship'.

- Good practice must always be in the context of 'Nothing About Us Without Us' (Charlton 1998), which helps combat isolation, loneliness and the stigma attached to the condition.

- This chapter has focused on the 'How', and not on the 'What', that underpins good practice, because the specifics of techniques and creative ideas can grow from solid values based on relational and person-centred foundations.

- Visit the Culture, Health and Wellbeing Alliance (CHWA) website at the URL supplied below for a more detailed look at the practice guidelines in the CHQF (2023).

References

APPG AHW (All-Party Parliamentary Group on Arts, Health and Wellbeing) (2017) *Creative Health: The Arts for Health and Wellbeing.* https://ncch.org.uk/appg-ahw-inquiry-report

Brooker, D. (2007) *Person Centred Dementia Care: Making Services Better.* London: Jessica Kingsley Publishers.

Brooker, D. and Latham, I. (2016) *Person-Centred Dementia Care: Making Services Better with the VIPS Framework.* 2nd edition. London: Jessica Kingsley Publishers.

Chaiklin, S. and Schmais, C. (eds) (1986) 'The Chace Approach to Dance Therapy.' In P. Bernstein (ed.) *Eight Theoretical Approaches in Dance-Movement Therapy.* Dubuque, IA: Kendall/Hunt.

Charlton, J. (1998) *Nothing About Us Without Us: Disability, Oppression and Empowerment.* 1st edition. Berkeley, CA: University of California Press.

Coaten, R. (2009) 'Building Bridges of Understanding: The Use of Embodied Practices with Older People with Dementia and Their Care Staff as Mediated by Dance Movement Psychotherapy.' Unpublished PhD thesis, Research Repository, University of Roehampton. https://pure.roehampton.ac.uk/portal/en/studentTheses/building-bridges-of-understanding

Coaten, R. (2022) 'Improvisatory Movement and Dance for Family Carers and Others.' In I. Parker, R. Coaten and M. Hopfenbeck (eds) *The Practical Handbook of Living with Dementia.* Monmouth: PCCS Books.

Coaten, R. and Warren, B. (eds) (2008) 'Dance – Developing Self-Image and Self-Expression Through Movement.' In B. Warren (ed.) *Using the Creative Arts in Therapy and Healthcare: A Practical Introduction.* (3rd edition, originally published in 2nd edition 1993.) London: Routledge.

Coaten, R. and Williams, S. (2016) '"Going far is returning": Dance movement psychotherapists find resilience and learning and call for more collaboration and dialogue.' *Dance, Movement & Spiritualities 3*, 1–2, 161–175.

Culture, Health and Wellbeing Alliance (2023) *Creative Health Quality Framework.* www.culturehealthandwellbeing.org.uk/resources/creative-health-quality-framework

Dewing, J. (2019) 'On Being a Person.' In D. Brooker (2019) (ed.) *Dementia Reconsidered, Revisited: The Person Still Comes First.* 2nd edition. London: Open University Press.

Greenblat, C. (2011) *Love, Loss, and Laughter: Seeing Alzheimer's Differently.* Guilford, CT: Lyons Pressan, Globe Pequot Press.

Hayes, J. (2011) *The Creative Arts in Dementia Care: Practical Person-Centred Approaches and Ideas.* London: Jessica Kingsley Publishers.

Innes, A. and Hatfield, K. (2002) *Healing Arts Therapies and Person-Centred Dementia Care.* London: Jessica Kingsley Publishers.

Killick, J. (ed.) (1997) *You Are Words: Dementia Poems.* London: Hawker Publications.

Kitwood, T. (1997) *Dementia Reconsidered: The Person Comes First.* Buckingham: Open University Press.

Kitwood, T. (2000) 'Introduction: Building Up the Mosaic of Good Practice.' In S. Benson (ed.) *Person-Centred Care: Creative Approaches to Individualised Care for People Living with Dementia* (Person-Centred Care series, published in *Journal of Dementia Care*). London: Hawker Publications.

Kitwood, T. and Bredin, K. (eds) (1992) *Person to Person: A Guide to the Care of Those with Failing Mental Powers.* Loughton: Gale Centre Publications.

Kontos, P. (2006) 'Embodied Selfhood: An Ethnographic Exploration of Alzheimer's Disease.' In A. Leibing and L. Cohen (eds) *Thinking About Dementia: Culture, Loss, and the Anthropology of Senility.* New Brunswick, NJ: Rutgers University Press.

NICE (2019) *Dementia. Quality Standard* (QS184). www.nice.org.uk/guidance/qs184

Parker, I., Coaten, R. and Hopfenbeck, M. (2022) *The Practical Handbook of Living with Dementia.* Monmouth: PCCS Books.

Rogers, C. R. (2004) *On Becoming a Person.* (First published in the UK 1967.) London: Constable.

CREATIVE ARTS PRACTICE

CHAPTER 3

A Creative Conversation about Arts and Memory

Jane Spiro and John Daniel

We are married partners whose partnership has been forged and strengthened through the creative arts. Both of us have loved poetry since childhood and share a love of writing, reading, performing and discussing poetry. John is also an artist working in acrylics, charcoal, pastel, pen and ink. My second 'art' is music, playing and performing the violin in quartets and trios. Both of us pursued these loved arts as adjuncts to careers in education. However, since 2019, John's experience of memory loss has bitten into his sense of safety and self, and in February 2023, this was diagnosed as mixed dementia.

This chapter shares the way in which dementia impacts on both John as an artist and me, Jane, as a partner and carer, making demands on our resilience as a couple. It centres on three conversations in which John is enabled to reflect on memory and the arts. The chapter considers the value of the creative arts as a site for wellbeing and concludes with insights into ways in which creativity can be nurtured alongside a cognitive impairment.

For several years before the diagnosis of mixed dementia in 2023, John had symptoms that were disturbing for us both. These included John's expressions of disorientation and unsafety whenever there were even small adjustments to routine, such as taking a different route home. Diversions from set plans, such as delays and late arrivals, triggered extreme anxiety and/or rage, often beyond what felt acceptable within a marriage. He also described feelings of rejection and loneliness in social settings that had long been safe and familiar; where he had once been a hearty participant in conversations, he became impatient and withdrawn.

In the light of these symptoms, the diagnosis of Mild Cognitive Impairment (MCI) in 2019 was a relief. First, I was able to understand these episodes of unreasonable rage and anxiety as symptoms of an illness rather than difficulties in a marriage. Second, I began to reach out for support, from friends and social services, gathering relevant information and reading the literature. For example, Talbot (2011), Gerard (2019) and Proffitt (2021) are daughters who supported a loved parent through the dementia journey. Though their stories are tender testimonies to love, they are also gruelling accounts of inexorable decline in a loved one, which no amount of loving care can halt. James (2008), Mumby (2012) and Andrews (2015) urge carers to validate the person with memory loss and corroborate their perceptions of the world, avoiding questions and contradictions, which exhaust and upset their relatives. The strategies are palpably successful; yet the carer, who was once in an equal partnership, is gifted with continuous curbing of their own conversational instincts. Supporting a loved parent is challenging enough, but as a changing dynamic with a life partner, it can come to feel like a very denial of the self.

In the midst of these very real challenges, as our conversations show, creative arts can be a safe and healing place, and a place of equality. Although we offer our personal observations and reflections as a couple, we are amongst many for whom this is also the perennial story of the quest for self-expression, the entitlement not only of gifted artists but of everyone – cared-for and carers alike.

Three conversations: art, poetry and memory
Conversation one: Poetry and memory

How has your subject matter changed
as a result of losing memory?
I focus on the immediate and now, such as landscape and shops – writing without the use of memory. Memory loss includes more acute observation as a kind of compensation. Sometimes I observe the details of my environment closely, or more tellingly, as a result.

When you read your own poems what do you notice?
When I look back at past poems, they seem enclosed by a memory that's now disappeared. Sometimes I'm not sure who wrote them, I am no longer the author. I realise poetry lurks in the immediate, what surrounds me at this moment. There is a kind of contemporaneity rather than recollected in the past.

What inspires you to write and has this changed
since your difficulties with memories?
From the beginning, and even now, reading inspires me. I think reading made me realise writing was an art form, and in some sort of way I wanted to imitate

that. I read more now but I forget it, so it's not quite so much a model – it was more of a model before. But I still value it as an inspiration and a stimulus for writing. I can't imagine writing without reading.

Has reading become more important than writing?

When someone loses their memory, to some extent they lose access to reality. I can't remember what happened this time last week. When I read I enter a densely fashioned world that is created by the author, and that in itself is a substitute. A writer always presents a bigger world for you than the one you inhabit.

Are there certain situations or conditions which help you to write?

All artists need an audience, either to read the work or to look at it. It could be that writing demands a fixity of memory, demands a lot of reference points that painting seeks to free itself from. It's useful to have people who look at your work, read it and respond. That's always important.

Are you revising work now, then, rather than writing new poems?

Yes. I think revision provides me with a foundation on which to build. Starting something brand new is difficult, and I do run out a bit. I don't perhaps have the multi-complexity of the original but it gives me a building block, something to start with. So it's become more important, more satisfying, or easier, than starting something new.

John wrote these poems when he was beginning to experience memory difficulties.

FORGETTING

I know you see still the colours
whether there is light in them, if they sing
against each other, if the earth is in them
or the air.

I know you are still the child
frustrated by suburbs, playing
the back lanes, finding
places of escape.
I know you remember still
the lines of poets, kingfishers and high seas,
ancient mariners, globed peonies,
and the ravelled sleeve of care.

But I do not know what it is you lose
as things become strange,
slide back day by day to zero,
the colours of our life
stripped back to white.
I stand against the tide,
hold memories in my hand, catch them
as they fall, carry them for safekeeping.

SPEAKING BACK
What I'd like to say to the nay-sayers
is yes
the leaps you said could not be made,
are yes, are made –

and when I slip my skin
you see its bright abandoned husk
and do not notice
I am no longer in it.

What I'd like to say
is yes.
we are continually wrong, I about you,
you about me, and that where I must go
is a leap from knowing
to not knowing, and you
must make the same leap too –

both of us, being brave,
from thinking we are right,
to wondering if we are wrong –

from holding a stone
to holding a question about space,
how it has evolved to be this.

Conversation two: Visual arts and memory

What do you feel about painting?

I make up painting as I go along. With painting it doesn't excavate the past in quite the same way. Also, abstract painting is very much to do with the present. It doesn't need the memory of trees or people. It is a contemporary act, maybe that's why it's become the dominant mode for me, because it's concerned with the present. Colours don't have a past. Colours have no memory or history, they are almost contemporary.

Has the way you look at paintings changed?
I look at things more carefully. I don't have the kind of panoramic sweep I had when I was younger, I concentrate on a specific spot; I become more detailed in my observation.

What about learning new things?
I am less inclined; I cling to the old methods because they are familiar and give me security whereas new methods are slightly threatening. For example, I use acrylics and paint mainly on paper, not canvas. Oil painting seems to be more of a paraphernalia now – turps, oil, canvas. I have used it in the past but I use acrylics now because they are simpler.

What inspires you to paint?
In a way, abstraction is more original than imitating reality and you experience greater freedom, liberty, choice of colour, shape, size, it's all in your hands, you can be more creative in painting than somebody who simply imitated a bunch of flowers or a vase. I feel memory loss in a way frees me in painting in a way it doesn't with poetry.

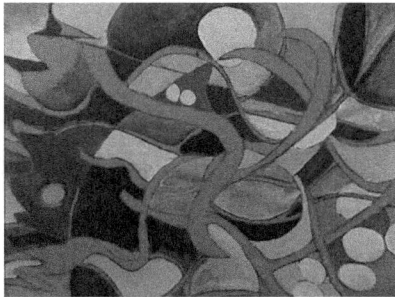

Figure 3.1 Res and Gold
PHOTOGRAPHY: JERRY MOERAN, STUDIO EDMARK, OXFORD.

Are there certain conditions which help you to paint now?
If I am writing or painting, it does help to have not only an appreciative audience but conditions which are supportive. I don't feel like writing under any circumstances, or painting under any circumstances. I don't think painting outdoors, looking at landscapes, is quite what you want to do with memory loss or getting older, because it seems less symbolic, less relevant and

somehow you feel you can do just as well without sitting outside in a field in the rain trying to paint.

Conversation three: reflecting on memory

What do you do to help your memory?

I keep a diary which is a record, and I do that partly to try and remember what's happened, to try and improve my memory, which I feel is slipping away. And the diary, with your help prompting me to remember, helps because the prompt brings back the memory and you can enlarge it.

The familiar, the known, the accustomed, are all reinforcing elements that help both writing and painting. The opposite, the strange, the alien, the new, the exotic, the unfamiliar, although they may once have been exciting, are now threatening. The unfamiliar becomes something you can't really incorporate because you can't remember where it's coming from or what it means. So I write and paint, not so much in the same place each time, but somewhere that's supportive.

Does painting, or writing poetry, make you feel less anxious and less lonely?

Ah yes, it's very absorbing. How happy you are depends on how successful the artwork is. You talk to the artwork and the artwork talks to you. If it's unsuccessful, if you're losing your memory, the artwork can become more important. If I think it's a good drawing, painting or poem, that would make me feel happy.

Do you feel proud of your work when it's finished?

If I think it's good, and if that's reinforced by other people. I don't think other people are the determining factor but I think they are important. People often articulate things I hadn't expected and quite surprise me. It enlarges your world, shows your work touches more points than I anticipated – it's bigger than your intentions.

Reflections of a carer and co-creator

These conversations suggest that when John is painting or writing he achieves a kind of healing. He returns to what is familiar and a place where he has mastery. The creative process acts as company, and his art and poetry reach out and speak for him. In this, he is not alone. Crutch, Isaacs and Rossor (2001) analyse the case of William Utermohlen, a 66-year-old artist, five years after a diagnosis of dementia. Over time, William's depiction of the human face becomes distorted, with elements missed out or in the wrong place. The researchers suggest this is a diminishing of artistic achievement and a manifestation of cognitive decline. Yet one could interpret the same data as testimony to the artist's enduring desire for self-expression. Though he solves the problem of perspective differently as his cognition changes, he is also using line and colour to shaft directly into his inner world.

Liggett and Wyatt (2022 p.292) describe Mary making decisions about her painting, choosing colour to match feeling rather than to imitate the outside world. She paints clouds pink because they 'cheer her up'. John, too, paints an imaginary pink road that winds through hills to disappear over a sunny horizon or the same road to the iconic industrial campaniles of Didcot Power station, now demolished. Many of his paintings are suffused with yellow and gold, as bursts of light. He paints a woodpecker, with gold paper pressed into its wings, and describes the sense of freedom and happiness when he paints without trying to represent or imitate the world.

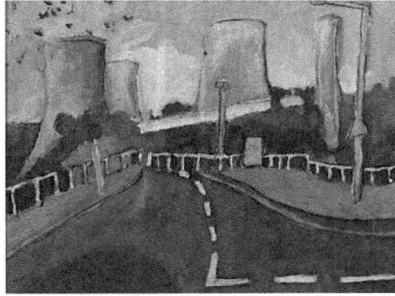

Figure 3.2 *Cooling Towers*
PHOTOGRAPHY: JERRY MOERAN, STUDIO EDMARK, OXFORD

William, Mary and John illustrate that being creative is an act of communication and a 'mechanism' for accessing feelings and memories. Matarasso (2012) would describe their changed management of shapes, colours, perspective as 'late style' and the artists themselves as 'tragic heroes, engaged in the final struggle for meaning' (*ibid*. p.60). In recognizing the work of elders as a source of value and beauty, we are 'rewriting the story of old age' (*ibid*. p.17).

Yet this 'final struggle for meaning' cannot happen in a vacuum. As a carer, there are multiple conditions I find it essential to provide so that John can continue with the creativity and engagement that nurtures him. These conditions include:

- ensuring he has dedicated space in the house to paint
- sourcing art classes and making sure he has transport to reach them

- cutting paper to size, rolling, packing and carrying it to his class
- inviting people to share poetry, art and music in our house
- creating opportunities for us both to read and perform poetry
- co-curating art exhibitions and gathering audiences from our shared communities.

The daily round of functional care is frustrating and relentless, and often feels self-denying. Yet through the arts, both of us arrive at a place of deep self-expression and resilience (Goulding 2018). John has learnt to listen as I play the violin in ensembles almost daily. Conversely, I appreciate and value his wonderful productivity as an artist daily. Through my brokering John's joining of various communities, he has been afforded other opportunities for participation in village life, which are also nourishing me.

Though no experience can be generalised from one couple to another, still our conversations suggest ways in which the conditions for creativity and self-expression might be nurtured for others too. Everyone has individual preferences and needs, so all the suggestions below require customising – not only to cognitive changes but also to changing feelings and moods.

- Set up a daily structured routine that builds in time for creative activities, ideally with a community of the like-minded, such as an art class or writing group.
- Find out what is available locally, such as a community choir, art exhibitions, art classes.
- Identify times in the day when the person is most alert/relaxed and schedule creative activity.
- Prepare and provide familiar surroundings and materials, such as drawing and writing, in known settings that are well lit by natural light.
- Prompt memory/recall about activities/methods/strategies by laying out the same paints, brushes, notebook for writing etc. and leaving them out as a reminder to return to work in progress to review, edit and revise.
- Ring-fence a quiet time to fulfil a task without interruption.
- Provide practical help to organise and administer creative activity, for example, help with formatting, filing and storing written work, getting information about suitable local groups and classes, arranging transport and buying suitable materials.
- Initiate and organise ways to share work and receive recognition, such as exhibiting paintings, reading or hearing one's poems read aloud in a group or to an audience.

- Keep a record of the creative outcomes (pictures, poems) so they can be used to return the person to the 'moment' as a prompt and to elicit reflection.
- Build on and support everyday creativity like cooking and gardening or parts of these activities that offer meaningful occupation and satisfaction.

These conditions provide the possibility of engagement, connection and agency. The anxiety, rage and alienation described at the start of this chapter have receded since John's diagnosis and since I have come to understand the sources of them. Whilst I have always recognised the calming and therapeutic power of the creative arts, what has changed is my realisation that the conditions for creativity must be proactively nurtured, as John's capacity to do so for himself changes. Art, music and poetry bring joy, they provide their makers with agency, a sense of self and self-worth and they offer something of profound value for all who are touched by them.

References

Andrews, J. (2015) *Dementia: The One-Stop Guide.* London: Profile Books.

Crutch, S. J., Isaacs, R. and Rossor, M. N. (2001) 'Some workmen can blame their tools: Artistic change in an individual with Alzheimer's disease.' *Lancet 357,* 2129–2133.

Gerard, N. (2019) *What Dementia Teaches You About Love.* London: Allen Lane.

Goulding, A. (2018) 'Setting the Scene: Older People's Conceptualisation of Residence and its Relationship to Cultural Engagement.' In A. Goulding, B. Davenport and A. Newman (eds) *Resilience and Ageing, Creativity, Culture and Community.* Bristol: Policy Press.

James, O. (2008) *Contented Dementia.* London: Vermilion.

Liggett, S. and Wyatt, S. (2022) 'The Magic of Paint.' In I. Parker, R. Coaten and M. Hopfenbeck (eds) *The Practical Handbook of Living with Dementia.* Monmouth: PCCS Books.

Matarasso, F. (2012) *Winter Fires: Art and Agency in Old Age.* London: The Baring Foundation. https://cdn.baringfoundation.org.uk/wp-content/uploads/2014/09/WinterFires.pdf

Mumby, T. (2012) *Conducting Well-Being with Dementia in the Family: New International Edition.* Abingdon: Trevor Mumby.

Proffitt, S. (2021) *The Lock-Picker: Dementia: A Love Story.* London: Palewell Press.

Talbot, M. (2011) *Keeping Mum.* London: Hay House.

CHAPTER 4

Songwriting with People Living with Dementia

Charlotte Cunningham and Mickey Bryan

Introduction

Charlotte Cunningham, Artistic Director of Turtle Key Arts, runs the Turtle Song initiative and has worked with composer and researcher Dr Mickey Bryan on three Turtle Song projects. This chapter begins with a brief overview of the importance of music for people living with dementia. It then describes the Turtle Song project, during which people living with dementia, carers, professional composers, directors and music students produce a song cycle over approximately ten weeks. Mickey Bryan draws on his ongoing research interviews with composers and music practitioners, which shows how they approach collaborative songwriting in dementia settings.

Why music?

Music is a unique mode of artistic communication which has the capacity to facilitate individual and collective emotional expression. For thousands of years, the production and diffusion of music could be found in countless cultures and social groups across the world. A person's musical journey may begin as early as in the womb, through detecting the melodic contours of the mother's voice and rhythmic heartbeat (Webb *et al.* 2015). During early infancy, evidence suggests that we assimilate many of the fundamental perceptual and even productive facets of musicality (Buren *et al.* 2021). Beyond childhood and throughout life, the presence of music is ubiquitous.

Music punctuates our lives, forges identities and fosters relationships integral to communal, participatory practices in which people come together to sing and play music. It enables us to communicate our deepest feelings, providing catharsis and joy. Hence, making and appreciating music is a near universal characteristic, and perhaps then, inherent to being human.

Music is now widely recognised and evidenced as a medium that can address and promote health and wellbeing throughout the human lifespan. The concept of 'music as medicine' has evolved in significant ways. As music therapy and community music practice have expanded during the 20th and 21st centuries, so has research into the benefits of music.

In this context, a multitude of benefits have been shown to vastly improve the lives of people living with dementia. Both active music-based interventions (MBIs) and receptive listening interventions have been demonstrated to stimulate various cognitive domains, and in some cases, improve or maintain cognitive functioning of people living with dementia. Studies support the use of MBIs for alleviating symptoms of impaired complex attention and executive functions (Särkämö *et al.* 2014), language processing (Dassa and Amir 2021) and perceptual motor functions (Braun Janzen *et al.* 2022). Music is particularly effective for improving memory functioning and encouraging autobiographical memory recall for people living with dementia (Thompson *et al.* 2021). There are many explanations for preservation of musical memory in people living with dementia. One is an overlap between areas in the brain associated with musical memory and those that remain relatively less affected by Alzheimer's disease (Jacobsen *et al.* 2015).

MBIs can ameliorate behavioural and psychological symptoms of dementia, including depression, anxiety and low mood (van der Steen *et al.* 2018), apathy (Holmes *et al.* 2006), agitation and irritability (Pedersen *et al.* 2017). Cumulatively, music can promote wellbeing, assist people living with dementia in everyday life and support carers (Cho 2018).

About the Turtle Song project

Turtle Song is a songwriting initiative for people living with dementia and their caregivers. It is primarily aimed towards people with mild to moderate dementia still living in their own homes. A group from a local community gather with a professional composer, a director and music students for a high-quality, challenging and enjoyable experience. Turtle Song takes place weekly over roughly ten weeks in arts venues or universities around the country, and the final session is shared in a performance space with invited family and friends and filmed. The project aims are to provide mental and physical stimulation whilst singing and working together as a community and to write and record a song cycle, composing brand-new material created by the entire group.

By the end of 2023, 66 song cycles had been completed in both the UK and internationally across 17 different locations and via Zoom during the pandemic. Having worked with more than 20 different composer/director teams and involved nearly 400 music students in Turtle Song, Turtle Key Arts are committed to sharing their model to inform best practice in the field.

Turtle Song project leaders work in partnership with local voluntary organisations and service providers to make contact with and recruit hard-to-reach people affected by dementia, isolation and depression. As participants write and perform their own song cycle, they improve and maintain cognitive pathways and raise self-esteem through empowerment (Särkämö *et al.* 2014, Baker and Stretton-Smith 2017).

Turtle Song is an intergenerational project, and the workshops are entirely accessible in terms of age and skill. An essential part of the process is the participation of young musicians, usually studying at local colleges and universities, who are instrumental in enabling people of diverse ages and experiences to learn from each other, challenge generational perceptions and barriers, and reduce stigma about dementia.

Delivering songwriting projects for people living with dementia

As part of ongoing research conducted by Mickey Bryan, a series of interviews took place to investigate the use of songwriting in dementia settings. Thirteen composers and music practitioners were interviewed to gain insight into their approach and to develop a toolkit that can be used in projects like Turtle Song.

Planning and structure

This overview of how these practitioners delivered their songwriting sessions shows that most practitioners devised their session plans in advance in order to provide a balanced structure to the session. However, strict adherence to the plan was considered less valuable than being able to adapt to changes to the order, timings and inclusion/exclusion of activities.

Every practitioner highlighted the significance of being *flexible*. One practitioner noted that 'planning is really important but being able to improvise away from the plan is *really* important'. As well as allowing successful activities more time to evolve, it was also noted that knowing when to stop an activity and move on to something new or take a break was essential.

Each practitioner typically structured their sessions in three parts, consisting of openers, songwriting activities and closers. It was noted, however, that the session's contents may change depending on how far along the project was. For example, rehearsing songs that had been composed throughout the project might be prioritised in later sessions, especially in advance of a final concert.

Openers and closers

Openers generally included physical and vocal warm-ups, hello songs and various musical games. Employing similar or the same openers each week helped establish a sense of familiarity, which benefitted the participants, cueing them to session expectations and surroundings. Physical and vocal warm-ups often adhered to a 'copy-back' style in which the practitioner modelled an activity for the participants to mimic. For physical activities, this included actions like rubbing hands, stretching and tapping along to music. Similarly, many vocal warm-ups used traditional call-and-response songs such as 'This Old Hammer'. These warm-ups were recommended for preparing the participants' voices and bodies for the rest of the session. 'Hello Songs' and 'Name Games' were particularly popular and used to receive and welcome each participant by name, as well as encourage social interaction in the group. A simple name game was described as asking each member of the group to introduce themselves, encouraging individuals to chant something like: 'My name's [insert name], it's nice to see you', in time to a musical accompaniment performed by the practitioner. The rest of the group would respond with 'He-llo [insert name], it's nice to see you.' Depending on the ability of the group, it could be extended in various ways, such as asking the participants to contribute something that they liked – for example: 'My name's [insert name], and I like tennis', followed by 'Her name's [insert name], and she likes tennis.' The objective for these activities was to instil a sense of fun and cultivate a good atmosphere in the room – hence, any activity must be accessible to all participants.

Closing activities were quite varied, although a common theme was to 'cool down' after more intensive activities through listening to a piece of performed music or singing a gentle, familiar song. Some practitioners opted to initiate a discussion reflecting on the session. In a similar vein, one practitioner used a creative activity in which participants used art materials on a big piece of shared paper to express their thoughts and feelings.

Writing lyrics

All practitioners started the songwriting process with lyric generation. Commonly, this would begin by initiating a group conversation to decide on a theme for the song. Once chosen, the practitioner would guide a conversation related to this theme. Stimuli, such as photographs, paintings and interesting objects, were sometimes presented to inspire the participants. Each practitioner stated how these discussions were effective for encouraging the participants to share personal stories from their lives. In addition to stimulating autobiographical memory recall, this method ensures that the lyrics are personally meaningful to each participant, allowing them to feel *ownership* of the song.

Several practitioners felt it was important to follow the participants' lead, to co-create rather than impose. One practitioner stated it was vital that 'everybody's voice is represented' and each participant 'had been listened to'. Practitioners would often pose questions to facilitate the process. Sensory-based questions relating to the song's theme were frequently used. For example, one practitioner described a song written about spring where they asked what kinds of things you might see/hear/smell during the season.

Once the lyrical ideas for the song were established and noted, many practitioners recommended splitting into smaller groups to write down sentences to form either a verse or chorus. Many noted that it was important to limit the number of lines to avoid it becoming too long and complex. Moreover, it was commented that some participants were less inhibited in sharing their creative ideas within a smaller group context.

Writing music

There were significant differences in how the practitioners approached composing music in their sessions. Some opted to set music to the lyrics written by the participants, composing the music away from the sessions and then rehearsing it with the group. Others preferred to facilitate as much participant-led musical composition as possible. Either way, every practitioner asked the group how they thought the music should sound. This could pertain to style, tempi, instrumentation and many other musical characteristics. These suggestions would inform how the practitioner should proceed in writing the music themselves or, alternatively, signified the initial phase of collaborative composition.

Once a general, verbal explanation of how the music could sound was decided upon, many practitioners sought to interpret and play a rough sketch of the description on their instrument. Typically, this might be simple, repetitive chord progression, adhering to whatever characteristics the participants had suggested (quiet, slow, melancholy – for example). The next step would be to 'invite a melody'. The simplest method would be for the practitioner to ask the group (not individual participants) if anyone had an idea for the melody. Then, using a line from the lyrics, a participant would sing an improvised melody over the practitioner's accompaniment. Once one participant had contributed, it was observed that others would often join in. However, if no melody was offered, then various contingency plans were suggested. Several practitioners recommended chanting the lyrics to a rhythm as a precursor for instigating melodic material. Others suggested a group improvisation, whereby everyone would sing simultaneously so as not to feel exposed. The practitioner would then listen out for melodic fragments to pick from.

The practitioners acknowledged that contributing melodies in this way was not always suitable for every participant, perhaps as a result of them being either less comfortable or less able to engage. As a result, they found other ways to involve these participants in the songwriting process. Typically, this involved posing compositional decisions for the participants to make. These might concern how the melody ought to evolve, such as asking if the second line should mimic the first or whether some variation should be introduced. More accessible, often binary, questions were specifically posed to participants who the practitioner had noted were more reserved. Every practitioner stressed the importance of everyone having had the opportunity to participate at a level that each participant was comfortable engaging in.

Using these strategies, practitioners would guide the participants through composing verses and choruses and any additional sections until eventually a fully formed song emerged. To help participants remember lyrics, many practitioners also used actions to accompany the words and made eye contact with non-verbal participants and those with hearing impairments. Many also invited the participants to dance, either from a standing or seated position, while taking account of mobility and safety. Multiple practitioners also handed out handheld percussion instruments for the participants to play along with. A final sharing for friends and family was considered a valuable way of concluding the project that provided participants with a sense of accomplishment, as well as joy for all involved.

Conclusion

Turtle Song is a model of good practice for enabling younger people living with dementia, and people with mild to moderate dementia and their carers, to engage in singing and songwriting. The chapter presents ongoing research into the methods and techniques used by practitioners to support people living with dementia in writing lyrics and music. Despite every practitioner having a slightly different approach, the importance of making and maintaining relationships is clearly paramount to fostering group cohesion, commitment and ownership over the creative process, as well as ensuring that each individual participates as fully as possible. Turtle Key Arts hope to continue to partner with many other musicians, practitioners and organisations to make their work accessible to more people across the UK and the world. All of the practitioners with whom we have worked are willing to share their experiences with those who are starting on this journey.

LEARNING POINTS

- Creating something *new* – there is a magic that comes from a group hearing the song they have composed for the first time. The overtly *creative* process and the sense of ownership and accomplishment that it imparts is somewhat unique to composing.

- Being flexible and pacing the sessions is key. Every group is different and therefore necessitates different ways of working. It is important to allow time to enjoy and explore activities and follow the participants' lead during the songwriting process. Similarly, moving things forward quickly can help maintain momentum.

- Everyone's 'voice' needs to be heard. Each person living with dementia, caregiver, composer, and student should be given an opportunity to contribute and express themselves in their own meaningful way.

- Turtle Song is a high-quality musical experience that promotes the personhood of people living with dementia who work creatively with professional composers and musicians in theatres and galleries.

References

Baker, F. A. and Stretton-Smith, P. A. (2017) 'Group therapeutic songwriting and dementia: Exploring the perspectives of participants through interpretative phenomenological analysis.' *Music Therapy Perspectives 36*, 1.

Braun Janzen, T., Koshimori, Y., Richard, N. M. and Thaut, M. H. (2022) 'Rhythm and music-based interventions in motor rehabilitation: Current evidence and future perspectives.' *Frontiers in Human Neuroscience 15.*

Buren, V., Müllensiefen, D., Roeske, T. C. and Degé, F. (2021) 'What makes babies musical? Conceptions of musicality in infants and toddlers.' *Frontiers in Psychology 12*, 5851.

Cho, H. K. (2018) 'The effects of music therapy-singing group on quality of life and affect of persons with dementia: A randomized controlled trial.' *Frontiers in Medicine 5*, 279.

Dassa, A. and Amir, D. (2021) 'The impact of singing on the language abilities of people with moderate to severe-stage Alzheimer's disease.' *Music and Medicine 13*, 3, 174–183.

Holmes, C., Knights, A., Dean, C., Hodkinson, S. and Hopkins, V. (2006) 'Keep music live: Music and the alleviation of apathy in dementia subjects.' *International Psychogeriatrics 18*, 4, 623–630.

Jacobsen, J. H., Stelzer, J., Fritz, T. H., Chételat, G., La Joie, R. and Turner, R. (2015) 'Why musical memory can be preserved in advanced Alzheimer's disease.' *Brain, 138*, 8, 2438–2450.

Pedersen, S. K. A., Andersen, P. N., Lugo, R. G., Andreassen, M. and Sütterlin, S. (2017) 'Effects of music on agitation in dementia: A meta-analysis.' *Frontiers in Psychology 8*, 742.

Särkämö, T., Tervaniemi, M., Laitinen, S., Numminen, A., *et al.* (2014) 'Cognitive, emotional, and social benefits of regular musical activities in early dementia: Randomized controlled study.' *The Gerontologist 54*, 4, 634–650.

Thompson, Z., Baker, F. A., Tamplin, J. and Clark, I. N. (2021) 'How singing can help people with dementia and their family care-partners: A mixed studies systematic review with narrative synthesis, thematic synthesis, and meta-integration.' *Frontiers in Psychology* 12, 764372.

Van der Steen, J. T., Smaling, H. J. A., van der Wouden, J. C., Bruinsma, M. S., Scholten, R. J. P. M. and Vink, A. C. (2018) 'Music based therapeutic interventions for people with dementia.' *The Cochrane Database of Systematic Reviews 2018, 7.*

Webb, A. R., Heller, H. T., Benson, C. B. and Lahav, A. (2015) 'From the cover: Mother's voice and heartbeat sounds elicit auditory plasticity in the human brain before full gestation.' *Proceedings of the National Academy of Sciences of the United States of America 112, 10, 3152.*

CHAPTER 5

The Artful Carer

Building Communities of Care Through Dance and Somatic Movement Education with People Living with Parkinson's and Their Caregivers

Melanie Brierley

Introduction

As a dance and movement artist in creative health, I specialise in working with people living with neurodegenerative conditions, including Parkinson's and dementia. Relevant for practitioners working with both populations, this chapter specifically focuses on my dance and movement practice for the Parkinson's community, described here as a process of artful care and a way to build Communities of Care. It illustrates the intricate ways in which movement, dance and Somatic Movement Education (SME) promote well-being in community groups through the use of artful and caring practices.

Parkinson's disease (PD) is a complex neurological condition involving movement disorders that bring significant physical change and mild cognitive problems, often leading to dementia (see Chapter 1). Generally, when nerve cells die or become impaired in PD, they lose the ability to produce dopamine, a chemical messenger or neurotransmitter. Normally, dopamine operates with other neurotransmitters to help coordinate nerve and muscle cells involved in movement. Without enough dopamine, this delicate balance is disrupted, and the hallmark symptoms of PD emerge (American Association of Neurological Surgeons 2024). These include tremors, rigidity, bradykinesia and impaired posture. Tremor is trembling in the hands, arms, legs and jaw. Rigidity is stiffness in the limbs. Bradykinesia is where movement slows down and disrupts gait. Impaired posture and coordination affect balance and lead to greater fall risk. In addition, physical changes in people living with dementia include visuospatial complications and difficulties when walking or standing from a seated position. Whereas the symptoms referred to above and responses to medication vary across the population, it is common, in my experience, for people with PD to experience flow disturbance (Eddy 2018). Understanding more about this idea of flow disturbance may greatly help the practitioner. It is key to all that I do in seeking to re-establish a sense of connection and flow for the person living with PD in and through movement, dance and SME. Family carers also encounter changes to their normal flow of life because they have less time to spend on themselves, socialise or find the energy and patience to meet the new demands of a caring role. Practitioners need to consider that groups can include partners/family carers; thus, attention needs to be drawn to the symptoms that impact these informal participants as well. For example, how to keep loved ones safe given gait problems, tremors and falls. Much of my work consists of facilitating carers to build on individual strengths, finding what could be described simply as coping strategies but which are much more than that, entailing high levels of practitioner experience, skill and knowledge. For example, carers share how dance supports relaxation and shifts mood when they are exhausted or at 'the end of their tether'. One carer identifies how sessions offer her 'emotional support' and 'time thinking about my own body', with another being 'less stressed at the end of the sessions, much calmer and able to cope.'

As a dance and movement artist in the PD community, I work with people's experiences of health and wellbeing. Holding safe spaces, being present and open to participants, and meeting with compassion what is spoken, seen and felt through shared body-based exchange requires me to find balance and remain steady through the encounters that land in my own body. In contrast to moments of joy and ease, I witness those of discomfort, anxiety and hopelessness, which may leave me feeling energetically depleted and saddened. In addition to reaching out for peer support and supervision, I embed care for myself through my practice to support my wellbeing and help me sustain my work. For all participants, including myself, I approach dance and movement practice as an artful carer.

Developing the artful carer

'Being an artful carer' is a term I use to describe how I purposefully promote the care of people living with PD by combining the art form of dance and SME as a therapeutic practice (Karkou and Sanderson 2006). I purposefully and sensitively focus on the parts of movement, dance and SME that I feel will support the person to experience themselves differently and to receive the therapeutic practices that might help them to move more easily, think through movement strategies, feel positive and manage daily life better.

My doctoral research (Brierley 2020) foregrounded the dance encounter as a connective and caring process. Thus, while I developed as an artful carer by more fully understanding the needs of people through shared dance practice in their homes, participants also discovered more about themselves and the artistry of movement and dance. This mutual exchange brought us closer to a shared understanding and helped form the basis of what could be described as a caring friendship. In group practices, this way of working is replicated with the intention that all of us can learn something from each other and create stronger bonds to build what I describe here as Communities of Care. I understand this term to refer to the process by which all group participants learn to care for themselves and each other through cooperation and co-creation. The practitioner no longer carries the sole responsibility for delivering or embedding practices of care; rather, participants have the agency to take care of themselves and other group members, which is in effect a form of empowerment. Each group grows, developing its identity and sense of community, born out of the shared creative, social and care-based experiences that take place within it and where dance supports self-esteem (Verlinden 2008).

Four key principles underpin my practice as an artful carer. I contend that Communities of Care flourish when these basic principles are applied. These are nurturing creativity, working with presence, ensuring safe and non-judgemental spaces, and developing compassion and empathy for self and others through movement practice. I now present a diagram of these key principles (see Figure 5.1), followed by a brief description of each. Additionally, detailed examples illustrate how they all link together in the practice of being an artful carer.

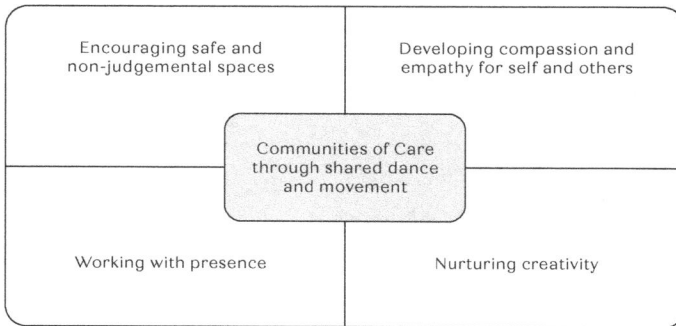

Figure 5.1 *Communities of Care through shared dance and movement*

Nurturing through creativity
Creativity is about working with the imagination, with the imagination taking us 'beyond and behind the everyday' and towards the 'active transformation

of experience' that makes the self visible (Levine and Levine 1999 pp.259–260). As an active transformation of experience, dance and SME have the potential to shift people's movements, feelings and self-perceptions. To this end, I use music and image-based/sensory vocabulary to support people's imaginations so that they can more fully connect with and experience their moving bodies. I talk and move at the same time within the group. As I am moving, I have a felt sense of my movement, and I describe it verbally, using imagery in my words that helps support others to move. At other times, if I feel that participants' movements are not coming through clearly, I stop and help break down the nature of the movement that we are exploring. Focused movement sequences support body awareness and enable participants to reconnect to a sense of self (literally and metaphorically). In movement, I facilitate a thinking process for the person such that they sense flow through sequential movement patterns. Together, we practise and learn skills and then express these skills creatively in movement to music.

Sometimes, I use touch with participants so that they have a felt sense of movement. For example, I might place my hands on a participant's shoulder blades, guiding small spiralling movements in their torso as support for their rotation. This is because I understand that if we want to recall movement, we need to know how it feels. Working through the 'felt' sense by using touch helps both mitigate diminished proprioception and support the motor symptoms of PD, which reduce flow experience in the body. Put simply, being able to remember how a movement feels is fundamental to its repeatability and accuracy. The kinaesthetic experience of dance enhances body-based engagement, with repetitive, creative, complex movements helping to integrate existing neural connections where there may be difficulties and enabling new ones to form (Farley *et al.* 2008).

Learned skills will then be incorporated into the next dance so that people can embody the movement, with the hope that some reconnection has occurred in the body through this exploration of the 'felt' sense of moving. The explorations surrounding this 'felt' sense are at the heart of my practice as an artful carer.

Safe and non-judgemental spaces

Dance groups are socio-communal places (Williamson 2009) and spaces of refuge (Fraleigh 1987) where participants feel safe, less anxious and accepted. As practitioner, I work with 'wide attention' and 'active listening', employing the skills of noticing and attention as essential facilitation processes for holding safe spaces (Fraleigh 2015). Safe and 'good enough' holding environments (Winnicott 1973) are created at the beginning and end of sessions, with participants either seated or standing. The group moves in the secure space of the circle, which also presents a performance area and a place to witness others moving. The following examples illustrate the use of the safe space offered by the circle. A participant moves tentatively across the dance space, passing a ball to another group member in a wheelchair. A carer holds their hands open and smiles mischievously, inviting their friend to dance in the movement circle. Partners connect through their fingertips in a delicate process of sensed and felt communication as they face each other in their chairs at the boundaries of the circle or work together whilst standing in the circle.

Working with presence: attending moment by moment to movement and dance

For Siegel (2007), presence is our capacity to be open to what is happening as it happens. The somatic psychologist Linda Hartley (1995) recognises that being present in our bodies is not only a form of awareness; rather, it is the first step towards being kind (and caring) to ourselves. Caring practices are promoted when I attend to my movement, slow down or listen closely to my breath. By modelling self-care, I encourage others to adopt similar ways of being so that ethical care for self translates into ethical care for others (Fortin, Vieira and Tremblay 2009). In the present moment, I learn to attune to participants' movements, connecting with their mood and energy. At the beginning of sessions, we take time to reconnect with ourselves, paying attention to our breath and touch, so that we can gradually open to working calmly. This is so important because many of the people in my sessions speak about their anxiety and fatigue. Working this way helps to calm the nervous system for us all, including me, which means that I then feel ready to engage with the people in the session and their different movement challenges.

Working with compassion

The foundations of caring communities emerge from a place of compassion. Like the motivational author Louise Hay (2004), I affirm loving, kind and accepting relationships with my body and encourage others to attend to themselves in similar ways. I use self-directed touch, with touch bringing attention and sensation to the body and a way to engage empathetically with ourselves. Self-directed touch is where people hold or touch their body parts to release weight and tension and enhance greater amplitude of movement. This may extend to moving in relationship with others, for example, supporting another's arm by letting it rest on top of your own helps to release tension in the musculature of the body and guide movement. Touch-based practice is about reconfiguring the person's own experience of their bodies in movement within the environment where the session takes place. Objects in the space and props, such as balls, sticks, bean bags and chairs, can provide haptic connection and feedback (hapticity relates to the sensed perception of touch as a means to support action).

Empathy

When people dance together, empathy emerges through shared body-based perceptions. Referring to Edith Stein, the phenomenologist Jaana Parviainen (2003) describes empathy as an act of knowing and one that entails a reliving or a placing of ourselves 'inside' another's experience. In a Chorley-based session (2022), a female participant and carer shared that, due to the complications of securing hospital appointments and spinal surgery for her partner with PD, their duet had been the most meaningful conversation of the week, with both expressing empathy through their non-verbal engagement. The following examples of movement and dance are also expressions of empathy explored by group participants.

Partners sit or stand closely, side by side. One person places their forearm underneath their partner's, creating connection and support for the hand, wrist and elbow. The person being supported allows their weight to land on the arm below. The partners breathe together, with the breath softening their bodies and helping them to feel one another's presence. Slowly, and with ease, the person in the supporting role starts to move their arm, listening and noticing the subtle responses of the other. Perhaps the movement becomes larger over time or they experience moments of hesitation and resistance to movement from their partner. Co-joined, the arms carve a pathway through space in this co-created caring and empathetic choreography.

Participants co-create short duets, combining spoken word with movement. In pairs, and as movers and witnesses, they take turns to speak and move, with roles later reversing. The empathetic exchanges are repeated with different partners so that the duets move around the dance space as shared communal acts of care:

> The Mover: I have been on a long and difficult journey (describe the journey through movement, for example, with high mountains and deserts). I'm so grateful for your help and support.
>
> Witness to the Mover: I see your long and difficult journey (mirror the journey). Let me help and support you on your way.

Final thoughts

After years of experience of working in this field, I have described above how I understand what being an artful carer is all about when I engage with participants receptively and responsively through SME and dance, out of which has emerged the idea presented here of helping build Communities of Care. In parallel, I have described four key principles that underpin all I do, giving a sense of how the complexity of this shared movement and dance experience creates subtle engagements of connection and flow, through which movement and creativity flourish. Without connection, flow is curtailed, and for people living with PD, this lack is fundamental to how they experience themselves. Connection thus gives back to the person essential aspects of themselves that may have attenuated through their condition. The practice identified helps people to look after themselves better, as I too look after myself through my practice, as well as engaging in creative supervision with experienced colleagues. This enables me to reflect on the challenges and success stories and to consider future opportunities for growth and development of myself and this remarkable work.

LEARNING POINTS

- Consider the four key principles and how they might impact your practice.

- How might you consider yourself an artful carer?

- How can you build Communities of Care in your practice?

- How might some fundamental aspects of connection and flow intersect with movement and dance in your sessions?

References

American Association of Neurological Surgeons (AANS) (2024) Parkinson's disease. www.aans.org/patients/conditions-treatments/parkinsons-disease

Brierley, M. (2020) 'Changing Perspectives Through Somatically Informed Dance Praxis: Reflections on One to One Dance and Parkinson's Practice as Home Performance.' Doctoral dissertation, University of Roehampton.

Eddy, M. (2018) Movement for people with Parkinson's. www.mixcloud.com/DrMarthaEddy/martha-eddy-movement-for-people-with-Parkinsons

Farley, B. G., Fox, C. M., Ramig, L. O. and McFarland, D. H. (2008) 'Intensive amplitude-specific therapeutic approaches for Parkinson's disease: Toward a neuroplasticity-principled rehabilitation model.' *Topics in Geriatric Rehabilitation* 24, 2, 99–114.

Fortin, S., Vieira, A. and Tremblay, M. (2009) 'The experience of discourses in dance and somatics.' *Journal of Dance & Somatic Practices* 1, 1, 47–64.

Fraleigh, S. H. (1987) *Dance and the Lived Body: A Descriptive Aesthetics*. Pittsburgh, PA: University of Pittsburgh Press.

Fraleigh, S. (ed.) (2015) *Moving Consciously: Somatic Transformations through Dance, Yoga, and Touch*. Urbana, IL: University of Illinois.

Hartley, L. (1995) *Wisdom of the Body Moving: An Introduction to Body-Mind Centering*. Berkeley, CA: North Atlantic Books.

Hay, L. L. (2004) *Love Your Body: A Positive Affirmation Guide for Loving and Appreciating Your Body*. London: Hay House.

Karkou, V. and Sanderson, P. (2006) *Arts Therapies: A Research-Based Map of the Field*. Edinburgh: Elsevier.

Levine, S. K. and Levine, E. G. (1999) *Foundations of Expressive Arts Therapy: Theoretical and Clinical Perspectives*. London: Jessica Kingsley Publishers.

Parviainen, J. (2003) 'Kinaesthetic empathy.' *Dialogue and Universalism* 13, 11–12: 151–162.

Siegel, D. J. (2007) *The Mindful Brain: Reflection and Attunement in the Cultivation of Wellbeing*. New York: W.W. Norton & Company.

Verlinden, J. (2008) We can nurture self-esteem, but how? www.communitydance.org.uk/DB/animated-library/we-can-nurture-self-esteem-but-how?

Williamson, A. (2009) 'Formative support and connection: Somatic movement dance education in community and client practice.' *Journal of Dance & Somatic Practices* 1, 1, 29–45.

Winnicott, D. W. (1973) *The Child, the Family and the Outside World*. London: Penguin Books.

CHAPTER 6

Creating and Sharing Poetry

Pat Winslow

Introduction

This chapter offers advice and guidance for creative arts practitioners interested in enabling people living with dementia to engage in poetry, outlines core skills and knowledge for collaborating with groups and encourages reflection and evaluation of poetry work.

Preparing

People living with dementia are not a single homogenous group; each person affected will have preferences for what they like to do, including reading poetry (or not), although offering poetry often prompts interest and engagement. We know that poetry, especially shared reading, stimulates emotions and feelings in the brain, promotes playfulness, flourishing and social connectivity, positively affects mood, behaviour and wellbeing and validates the personhood of people living with dementia.

You don't have to know all there is to know about poetry to run a good session. You don't even have to be a brilliant poet. You need a passion for it, though. You may already have favourite poems and poets, but do continually seek to broaden your reading. Take *The Poetry Cure* (Darling and Fuller 2005) or visit *The Poetry Pharmacy* (Sieghart 2017), as you will be meeting and working with people with a diverse cultural heritage.

Find poems in translation for bilingual participants or those who speak their mother tongue fluently, perhaps starting with *In Person 30 Poets* (Astley and Pearce-Robertson 2008), an anthology of poems in many languages in a parallel-text format and two CDs of authors mainly reading in varieties of English. These include Benjamin Zephaniah, who melds Birmingham and Jamaican, and Jackie Kay, who was brought up in Scotland. Palestinian poet

Taha Muhammad Ali reads in Arabic and then re-inhabits each poem as it is read in English by his translator Peter Cole.

Be curious – not just about other people but about language in general. Learn how to say hello and thank you in the languages of people you meet and greet. It can make a world of difference.

Be adventurous and, crucially, an active listener so that you learn from people living with dementia, perhaps by reading first-hand accounts such as those by Wendy Mitchell (2022) and from poets who draw on conversations with care home residents to create poems (Killick 2018), and shadow other Creative Practitioners if you can.

Group work

When creating poetry with a group, remember that closed questions yield yes/no answers whilst open questions create the opportunity to respond uniquely. People may feel anxious about poetry. 'It's not for me', they might say. 'I don't understand it.' Go in with a flip chart and lots of decent pens but explain that you are not expecting anyone to write unless they want to. Be their scribe. Not having to worry about handwriting and spelling creates freedom for sharing thoughts and ideas. Once you have covered the pages with words, help the group edit by cutting the words up and moving them around on a table or on the floor. The group poem is one of the most empowering ways to engage people.

Understanding group dynamics is vital. No two groups are the same. Even the same group might vary from week to week. Try to be sensitive to the needs of people. Sitting in a circle, so everyone can see, hear and listen to each other, encourages turn taking and working together. Having a variety of stimuli at your disposal makes it easier to manage attention spans. Equally, people need quiet to think. Finding a memory or a word isn't like flicking a light switch. It's more like reeling a fish in from the bottom of a lake. If what comes up is an old boot, celebrate that. Quirky poetry is sometimes the most inventive. Never shut up a dominant person; just thank them for their contribution and then show a keen interest in other people's contributions.

Planning

When planning a session, I like to have a theme. I choose a handful of poems and print readable copies using a font like Arial in size 14 or above. If I've been working with a group for a while, I'll ask them to choose a topic each week. In addition to poems, I'll create a playlist. This creates a positive atmosphere of anticipation and reminds people of what we are here to do. I may use pictures and objects that relate to the theme and will have my flip chart to hand. We will always make a group poem at some point to bring everything together.

Prepare your session on paper or a tablet and in your head. Organise your materials and bring *everything*. Nothing will ever go exactly to plan, and you may occasionally need a Plan B. One session I ran was about owls. I had a playlist of night sounds and well-known songs about moonlight. There was a toy owl you could blow into to create an eerie hoot and a handful of poems. I also had Plan B, just in case.

A quarter of the way through, I was just about to launch into George Macbeth's 'Owl' (2017).

D started shouting, 'No! No! No owl! No!' I asked what was wrong. 'An owl means death! It always does.' She began listing all the people who had died.

'It's true', said J. 'My father saw an owl up a pole and he went into hospital and there was an owl there too.'

'Yes, an owl means death', someone else said. In a matter of seconds, D had us on the edge of a precipice. Plan B was hastily implemented, but not until we'd listened to a calming track from my playlist.

Looking back on my journal, I can see several factors that should have been clear warning signs:

- I was late and disconcerted because of a four-car pile-up.
- The room was hot, and people were tired.
- There were 17 participants, not the usual 10–12.
- The activity coordinator was distracted and kept disappearing.
- M kept falling asleep and waking up shouting that she wanted to go home.
- J was hungry.
- There were no staff to help.

With that in mind...

Check-in

Who's present, who's missing, how are people feeling? How are *you* feeling? If in a care home, how is the activity coordinator today? Is an extra level of support needed? Be aware of energy levels, mood, comfort, lighting conditions, temperature and whether people can see and hear each other, and resolve issues if you can.

Games and exercises

A warm-up is essential. I favour circular call-and-response games that remind us of each other's names – I'm Brenda and I like bread; I'm Mahmoud and I like mangoes. We might act out eating the food: great for getting everyone moving as well as thinking about words. I actively listen and note who's quiet and perhaps not very confident and who is apt to dominate.

Take into account individual strengths and needs so everyone can access and enjoy the session. Start by reading a handful of poems together, which is supportive of less confident readers and helps the group cohere. If members of the group do not have severe dementia, one or two people can be invited to read solo. Although everyone has printed copies, I might also ask people to listen to poems with their eyes closed, if it's appropriate, and to notice the rhythm and meaning. Allow space for each poem to sink in. Invite feelings and thoughts. What were people's favourite lines? 'Why?' is a bread-and-butter question.

One week, I followed this up with kitchen utensils stuffed inside big woolly socks. Everyone had a go at describing what the shapes felt like as they passed them round. Once the objects were revealed, we added other descriptions – textures, sounds, smells. An old rotary kitchen whisk became a percussion instrument, which in turn became a cue for a song. Music tuned us into rhythm and emotions.

Listen out for something that can provide a spark. You will know it when you hear it. Other people may react to it, too. Create a moment for the spark to ignite further. Repeat the line. Write it on your flip chart. Invite rejoinders.

Here are three examples that sparked wonderful group poems:

I've got a forgettory.
Hands can be a prayer, a cup, begging.
Falling in love is like jam tarts.

The group poem

The next stage involves gathering words on the flip chart. With so much energy and enthusiasm, the real challenge for the scribe is to be quick enough to catch what everyone is throwing into the pot. Do remember, your job is to ask questions and listen, not to advise or correct. Don't interrupt silences when people are thinking. If people do get stuck, throw in another question.

The aim is to produce a working draft. Gather the lines and read them back. Encourage people to shift the order, move words about, explore what's being said and add further lines. Read everything back again. Check the rhythm. Explore the sound of what's being said. Allow the group to sculpt the poem till they are happy with it. When it's finished, find a title.

The poem belongs to the whole group, so credit everyone by writing their names at the bottom of the paper (but ask for their consent to do so).

I always give everyone a printed copy to keep the following week.

Here's one I made with residents of Chilterns Court, Henley, during the Making of Me, led by The Courtyard, Hereford, one of four projects that made up a three-year arts in care homes programme (Dix, Gregory and Harris 2018). (The residents haven't been credited here to preserve anonymity.)

Misadventure
Going out to sea,
rowing out to sea,
seven cats in a boat
with a woman –
sinking!
Cold, wet and horrible.
Cats don't like water.
She's a wicked woman.
Swim!
Swim ashore, pussy!
You can do it!
Don't worry about
how many miles.
Ashore, seven cats running
to the driest point in the sun.

Person to person

Individual poetry creation is quieter and more intimate. The last thing you want to do is overwhelm someone.

If you are visiting a room in a side ward, always knock before entering. Respect personal space. Introduce yourself. Say why you are there. Ask if it's OK to chat for a while – if you may pull up a chair and sit down. Bring and read a printed copy of a poem – and let it sink in for a bit. This is a conversation. Don't be afraid to ask questions. 'Does the poem remind you of something? Do you want to share that?' Ask if it's OK to write down what they are saying to make a poem from it. The minute you have put the possibility of poetry into someone's mind, their attention to language can shift. Rhythm is inherent. Pay attention to someone's speech patterns. Don't change what they're saying. Just write it down as you hear it. Remember – active listening. Always. Be open to magic.

When they've finished telling you, read it back. Read it with the same generosity you used when sharing the printed poem earlier on. Treat the text as something of value. Ask the person if they want to change anything. Try not to impose your opinions but do say what's working for you. And tell the person why.

Here's a remarkable piece of work by a patient in Witney Community Hospital, who participated in the award-winning Oxfordshire Community Hospitals Creating with Care arts programme.

The Nine Lives of a Cat

1

Something very like a trap.

2

You could hang it.

3

A big barn and a jump too far.

4

Cut up on the trailers.

5

Have a rabbit (we're over half-way there now).

6

Caught by a ferret.

7

Found in a vat of cider.

8

A storm, a wind took it out on the prairies where it blew about and caused havoc.

9

A ride in a carriage in the distance.

This evolved from a sustained effort on G's part. After each statement, there was a pause whilst she considered the next possibility that came into her mind. She was living with advanced dementia, from what I could tell, but her narrative thread was absolutely clear, and she never wavered.

We can't underestimate the power of creativity. If the right word has escaped, another will be found. My own stepfather told me about a 'grey whispery thing' that used to come past his window. He didn't mention the tail or the silence of his room, but it's all there in the conjoinment of grey and whispery. And doesn't whispery sound like whiskery? I was in no doubt he was talking about a squirrel.

Poetry defies labels. When a woman described as 'non-verbal' responded to Seamus Heaney's 'St Kevin and the Blackbird' (1996) with a detailed memory of her cats, it felt like a miracle had taken place. There's something about Heaney's intensity of language and the absolute simplicity of his telling. The poem is visual. We can see the blackbird laying its eggs. We can sense Kevin's endurance, feel wonder that a bird might make a nest in a man's hand. Heaney's poem opened a door that day and gave access to a memory that had been forgotten. The woman was completely herself when she was describing her cats so completely in the moment of memory; there was no indication that she was living with dementia.

Reflecting and evaluating

You will, of course, learn so much more about relating to people living with dementia and yourself as a facilitator if you pay attention and keep a journal to record what's said and done in a session and review and reflect on what you did, how you felt, what you learnt and what you will do next time.

We can evaluate the impact of poetry on a person in many different ways using many different measures (Chapter 15 includes references to reflective practice models that can be used for this purpose), but we should always observe and record participants' responses to poems.

Given the isolation experienced by people living with dementia, it is also enormously valuable to measure the extent to which poetry sessions enable people to interact with each other. When people start listening to each other and asking each other questions, that's a sign that social engagement is taking place on a meaningful level. Especially the listening.

It's good to end a session with a group discussion in a circle to mark the end of the activity and to provide space and time for reflection and for you to gather feedback. Start with questions that people can easily answer and then present those that require more thought, for example, 'What did you find the most difficult today?' or 'What was the most surprising thing you discovered about yourself?' Shortening or rephrasing questions and prompting memory can help, for example, 'What was difficult about the poetry we did today?' Sometimes responses are spontaneous. Someone whose memory is quite fragile telling you 'I feel like me' or that their confidence is coming back, that they feel more alive and more real, shows poetry is helping them make connections with emotions and feelings.

Final thoughts

Without reflecting on and evaluating my work and a substantial body of notes, I wouldn't have been able to write this chapter. Do make it a regular part of your practice to share insights with peers and colleagues if you have them, respecting the people you're working with at all times by anonymising material shared. Their generosity should never be abused.

LEARNING POINTS

- Respect the person: find out a little about who you will be sharing and/or writing poetry with and source poems that are likely to appeal to their personal experience and interests.

- Plan around a theme that provides opportunities for everyone involved to participate, even if they choose not to.

- Don't rush. Check in to find out how people are feeling and provide space and time for a warm-up, introductions and a clear ending.

- Prepare more material than you think you will use; you may have to improvise if the participants respond positively to a particular topic or change direction in response to disinterest or distress.

- Always make notes, evaluate and reflect on your work and enhance your learning, and the learning of others, by regularly sharing this process with peers and colleagues.

References

Astley, N. and Pearce-Robertson, P. (2008) *In Person 30 Poets*. Hexham: Bloodaxe Books.

Darling J. and Fuller, C. (2005) *The Poetry Cure*. Hexham: Bloodaxe Books.

Dix, A., Gregory, T. and Harris, J. (2018) *Each Breath is Valuable: An Evaluation of Arts in Care Homes Programme*. London: Baring Foundation. https://baringfoundation.org.uk/resource/each-breath-is-valuable-an-evaluation-of-an-arts-in-care-homes-programme

Heaney, S. (1996) 'St. Kevin and the Blackbird.' In S. Heaney (1996) *The Spirit Level*. London: Faber & Faber.

Killick, J. (2017) *Poetry and Dementia: A Practical Guide*. London: Jessica Kingsley Publishers.

MacBeth, G. (2017) 'Owl.' In K. Towers (ed.) (2017) *Ten Poems About Birds*. 2nd edition. Nottingham: Candlestick Press.

Mitchell, W. (2022) *What I Wish People Knew About Dementia: From Someone Who Knows*. London: Bloomsbury.

Sieghart, W. (2017) *The Poetry Pharmacy: Tried-and-True Prescriptions for the Heart, Mind and Soul*. London: Particular Books.

CHAPTER 7

Maggie May: Co-Creating a Play about Adapting to Life with Dementia

Nicky Taylor, Rosa Peterson and Frances Poet

Introduction

We'd like to tell you a story. It's not about someone extraordinary or privileged but someone leading an ordinary life, like many of us. And it's a story many families might find familiar, because our central character has dementia. In this chapter, we will share how our play *Maggie May* developed, and how the three of us (Nicky, Rosa and Frances) brought different perspectives and skills to the project. And whilst *we're* telling you this story, it's actually the story of many more people – some who would define themselves as artists and many who wouldn't – who contributed in different ways over five years to co-create this piece. Some of them got to see the final version and some sadly didn't. All of them made a profound impact on how the story was shaped and shared.

Dementia on stage

From Shakespeare's King Lear experiencing violent outbursts linked to Lewy body dementia (Escolme 2018) to Florian Zeller's *The Father*, in which a frightening, truth-twisting reality disrupts relationships between an older man and those around him (Chansky 2023), characters with dementia are often portrayed as a burden or a stigmatised 'other' with experiences to be pitied or feared (Basting 1998, 2006, Zeilig 2012). While plays about dementia may have created more awareness, it is possible they have also created more fear, with few moving beyond stereotypical tropes of loss and decline. This may be in part because plays about dementia are written by those left behind: a son, daughter or partner who has experienced the challenges of caring and ultimately the loss of the person they love. These stories are incredibly important, but Nicky, who instigated and leads the theatre and dementia programme at Leeds Playhouse, began to ask: what if a play about dementia had a different starting point and could be guided by people who are living with dementia?

> Working creatively taught me just how brave and bold people with dementia can be, but I hadn't seen any plays which represented this. I wanted to see a character who adapted to life with dementia as well as possible and could ultimately offer audiences some hope. There was also a need for a piece about the experience of dementia written supportively and sensitively *for* people diagnosed with dementia, as target audience members. To the best of our knowledge, this had not been done before.

Rationale for a different story

And so we commissioned *Maggie May* in 2017 as part of 'Every Third Minute: A festival of theatre, dementia and hope at Leeds Playhouse', which was curated by people living with dementia and their supporters.

In line with the festival's co-production ethos, we wanted the play to highlight just how much people with dementia, like Maggie, have to offer. They remain a part of the daily lives of their families, fulfilling roles as partner, parent, friend and confidante.

Rosa is one of these people, who advised on the process of making *Maggie May* and became a curator of Every Third Minute festival, making decisions about programming and presenting work on stage about the experience of dementia. Rosa has vascular dementia:

> Every experience of dementia is different. Some of us can do a lot and some of us can't do as much. Lots of people think you can't do anything if you have dementia. I try to do as much as I can. (Taylor, Peterson and Poet 2020 preface)

Starting the process

We wanted to tell the story of an ordinary woman living in Leeds, amongst a network of family, friends, social and working connections, who was experiencing recognisable challenges in adapting to life with dementia in the first year after diagnosis. This play would be a slice of life and not end in death. Crucially, we wanted this play to be accessible and welcoming to audience members living with dementia.

Writing in 2020, Frances said:

> I was more than a little intimidated by the brief. My dear dad had dementia
> and there was not much that was positive about our experience as a family,
> supporting him through it. I didn't know then to seek out groups where he
> could meet other people with the condition. I didn't know it was possible to
> find creative, nurturing spaces where he could make significant contributions.
> So it was with trepidation that I accepted the commission to write *Maggie
> May*. I need not have worried. From the moment Nicky introduced me to
> the extraordinary people living with dementia who were connecting with
> the Playhouse in various ways – funny, open, interesting and resilient peo-
> ple – I knew I could write the play. And so, Maggie was born: a feisty, funny,
> no-nonsense Leeds woman who carried the spirit of all these people who
> had inspired me and been so generous in the way they shared their stories.
> (Taylor, Peterson and Poet 2020 preface)

The whole process was rooted in generosity, as Rosa reflects without hesitation, considering why she got involved:

> To help other people, by talking and focusing on what they can do, not what
> they cannot do. Telling those stories can make people realise that we *can* do
> things and maybe the play might make people think differently.

Building relationships, gathering ideas

We began in summer 2017 with a week of research and development meetings at Leeds Playhouse. Around 20 people of different ages and ethnicities,
with different types of dementia, spoke openly about their experiences of
dementia. Frances recalls:

> But *Maggie May* wasn't written simply by meeting a group of people and
> incorporating their stories. Nicky set up a highly collaborative development
> process in which people living with dementia, and their supporters, had a
> significant dramaturgical input at every stage. (Taylor, Peterson and Poet
> 2020 preface)

We built trust, tested ideas and gained new perspectives, often carefully
navigating the different experiences of people with a diagnosis and their
supporters. Frances positioned herself as a keen learner in order to soften
any power dynamics between professionals and people with lived experience.
One contributor spoke of their initial reluctance to join a dementia support

group. He told his wife he intended to sit at the back and remain invisible but realised this plan was unworkable when he arrived to discover the chairs arranged in a circle. This man, once so shy, made the greatest of contributions to our artistic discussions in these early stages, offering many thoughts, ideas and jokes. He truly embodied the concept of the possibility for growth after diagnosis. These early contributions helped build the spirit of the play, and Frances developed an early draft.

First chance to share

We hosted a rehearsed reading of a draft script during Every Third Minute festival early in 2018 for an audience of 50 people affected by dementia. This was a pivotal moment to see how the play might resonate with our target audience. Frances recalls:

> In the first reading, I was sitting behind a man living with dementia who was vocal in his enjoyment of the jokes and songs. It was suggested at the beginning that he might not manage to stay for the second half – but he did, and at the moment in which Maggie explains to her son that though she might not always remember his face or name, her heart will always know him, this audience member turned to his wife and gave her a nod to say, 'That's how I feel about you.' (Taylor, Peterson and Poet 2020 preface)

Sharing the script with its intended audience, we were able to co-develop approaches to accessibility, the use of music and how the humour and emotional scenes might land. We discarded a distracting 'neighbour-in-need' narrative and instead allowed Maggie to have a positive impact on her son's girlfriend, allowing a tighter focus on the core family unit.

Collaboration and refinement

In 2019, we gathered with a group of actors to work through the latest draft alongside some new collaborators affected by dementia who had become involved in Leeds Playhouse life in the interim. This is the reality of making work about dementia: there will always be new people diagnosed, new stories to learn from and new perspectives to include. People with different sub-types of dementia found that their experiences varied, especially in a representation of Maggie experiencing an acute delirium. This was difficult to navigate and had to be addressed openly with collaborators with dementia to find a resolution. We acknowledged the contradictions in the condition and discussed typical experiences of people with different diagnoses, and collaborators agreed between them that if what was represented felt true for some of our contributors and for Maggie's character, then we should include it. Rosa feels this was important:

> It was us telling our stories, not other people, it's first-hand experience, we're living it.

Solidarity between collaborators with dementia and our creative approach meant there was safety in disagreement. A focus on learning more about each other's experiences and finding solutions became our natural approach. Frances responded to concerns by softening the representation of extreme distress while maintaining authenticity, cutting one of the more aggressive moments of Maggie directly addressing the audience. We also shifted the position of the interval to allow the audience to see Maggie in a more positive place before the break. Nicky checked in one-to-one with collaborators to ensure that they felt their voices had been heard and were comfortable with how Maggie's story was developing.

Preparing for performance

In February 2020, the cast for *Maggie May* gathered alongside director Jemima Levick, set, lighting and sound designers, and people living with dementia who had supported the process to reach this point. Rehearsals started with an introduction to what dementia is and how it feels to live with it so that the professional team could learn the importance of lived experience and how it grounded the play. Bonds formed between actors and the people whose experiences they were representing. Throughout the rehearsal process, people affected by dementia, including Rosa, watched specific sections of the play to support the delicate task of finding the balance between truth and drama in the story and, crucially, avoiding frightening people. With only minor script changes needed during rehearsals, the energy of collaborators with dementia went into shaping the representations of hallucinations and moments of acute confusion with members of the creative team. For some, this was emotionally tiring, while others felt buoyed by seeing their experiences being given dedicated time and a sense of importance. Again, checking in with a chat after rehearsal sessions was vital to offer opportunities to raise concerns outside the group and to take ongoing care of people offering their lived experience.

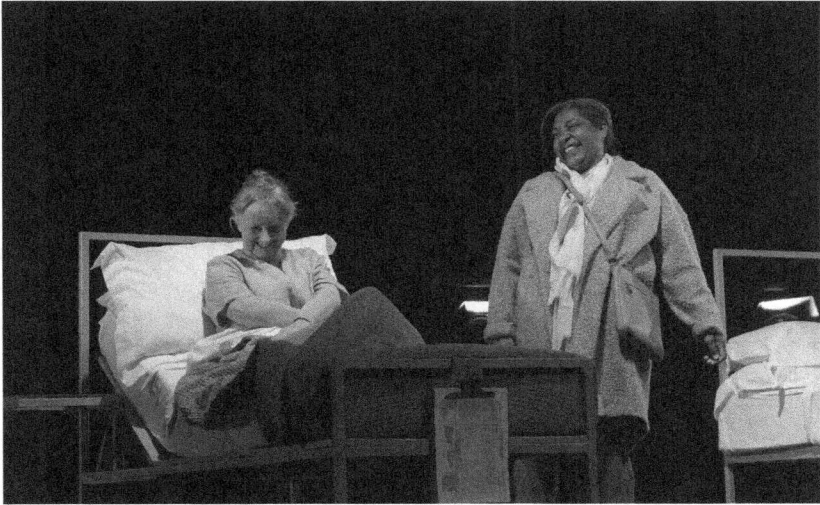

Figure 7.1 Maggie (Eithne Browne) and best friend Jo (Maxine Finch), 2022 production of Maggie May at Leeds Playhouse
PHOTOGRAPHY: ZOE MARTIN

Importance of production design

Working alongside collaborators with dementia, we co-developed techniques that aimed to help people stay connected to the play. For example, short narrative reminders about people and place appeared in text on caption boxes, as well as being voiced aloud by Maggie, guiding audiences into each scene and helping them to stay oriented as the scene progressed. A specific colour palette was chosen for each character's costumes, making it easier for audience members to stick with who's who. For example, Maggie's husband Gordon always wears brown. The sound design and the use of music acted as a supportive attention grabber and a welcome interlude from dialogue. Audience members were invited to sing along to familiar tracks, with lyrics provided on caption boxes on the stage, and this active participation aimed to sustain engagement and concentration. With all this in place, we felt confident to welcome audience members with dementia to all our performances.

Arrival of COVID-19 and its impact

We had just opened the second preview of *Maggie May* when the UK government told theatres to close due to the threat of COVID-19. This was a heartbreaking moment. *Maggie May* wasn't able to open until its premiere at Leeds Playhouse in May 2022, before touring to Queen's Theatre Hornchurch,

London and Curve Theatre, Leicester. Of course, the narrative of how our society values older people and people with dementia could not have become more relevant, as these groups were disproportionately affected by COVID-19 (Tuijt *et al.* 2021), and it felt more important than ever to highlight the value and contribution that people with dementia make to society. Our team was acutely aware that some people with dementia who had been involved early on in the process were unable to be part of celebrating the play's impact on audiences. *Maggie May* was extremely well received in local and national reviews, including a five-star review in The Stage, and generated extremely moving, relevant and energising audience feedback. As Rosa said:

> I hope when people see it, it makes them more understanding and more patient. (Taylor, Peterson and Poet 2020 preface)

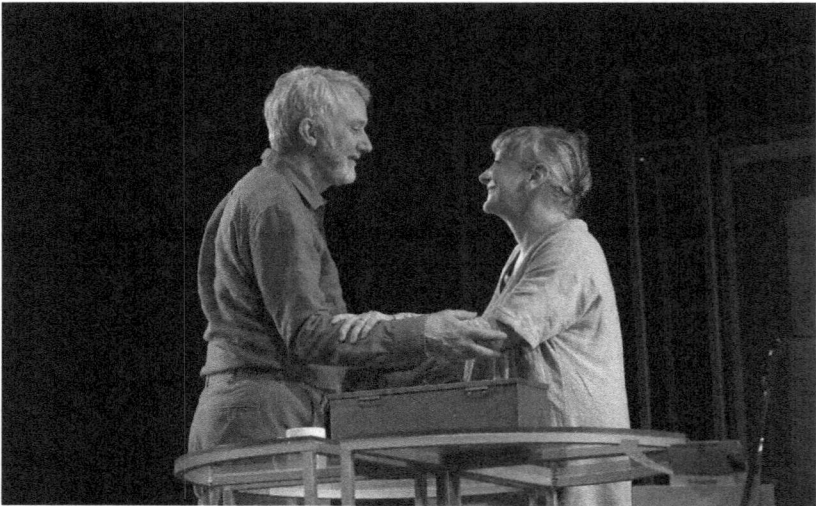

Figure 7.2 *Maggie (Eithne Browne) and husband Gordon (Tony Timberlake), 2022 production of Maggie May at Leeds Playhouse*
PHOTOGRAPHY: ZOE MARTIN

Learning from the process

Maggie May reinforces what's possible when we co-create and value voices that are less often part of the conversation, and it resonated with audiences in different ways. In total, 3500 people saw our play, and current or former carers reported in post-show feedback that they found the scene between Maggie and her son particularly moving. When Maggie explains that even if she forgets his name or face, her heart will always know him, this highlighted how much insight and agency people with dementia may have in ways that are not often dramatised.

> Beautiful and uplifting portrayal of how a dementia diagnosis can impact the whole family.

> Really inspiring to also see how the play has been made accessible for people with dementia and reaffirms theatre's crucial role as a central hub to connect communities. (Audience member)

For people with dementia, being offered a balanced story of adapting and coping, where a character with dementia remains resolutely herself throughout, was a welcome change.

> Thank you for showing a realistic portrayal of how Alzheimer's can affect the person and the family, friends, well written, beautifully acted. (Audience member)

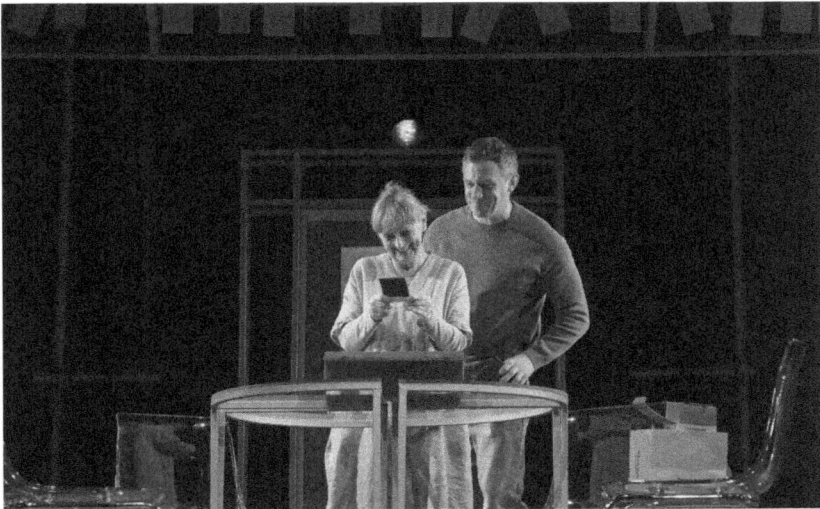

Figure 7.3 Maggie (Eithne Browne) and son Michael (Mark Holgate), 2022 production of Maggie May at Leeds Playhouse
PHOTOGRAPHY: ZOE MARTIN

Where are we now?

There are many more stories to tell, and there will be more individuals and families affected by dementia who will benefit. Nicky's long-term plans for building on this work are to co-produce a centre for theatre and dementia practice. She is currently running a study creatively engaging people with dementia in the earliest stages of imagining what such a centre might be.

Rosa continues her creative contributions in Leeds Playhouse activities, though this has felt more difficult since the frightening reality of the pandemic:

> I'm scared of catching the bus now, and it limits what you can do. Instead, I have to get a taxi, which means I do less than I did before, because it's harder to organise.

Maggie May was selected as a finalist for the prestigious Susan Smith Blackburn Prize, the oldest and largest playwriting prize honouring women and writing for the English-speaking theatre. This brought the play international recognition and reinforced our intention for the project to bring artistic excellence alongside a local community-centred process. It was gratifying to know that Maggie's story felt as resonant to a judging panel based in America as it did to us in Leeds.

Since the play was published, amateur theatre companies have acquired the rights to stage their own productions of *Maggie May* across the UK and America. Indeed, of Frances's many published plays, none have had comparable uptake with amateur groups as *Maggie May*. It's clear that the story holds great resonance. It is thrilling to see that the Leeds Playhouse model and Maggie's message of hope after diagnosis will be reaching people in community centres and village halls over the years ahead. It may find someone at the very moment they need to hear that there is a way to live hopefully with dementia.

LEARNING POINTS

- Acknowledging and attending to power dynamics is a vital part of creative collaboration, and humility and openness are essential. How are you strengthening relationships to build trust that will help move you from being strangers to working together as collaborators?

- Don't rush the process. Valuing the contributions of people with dementia takes time, and it alters the stories we tell. How have you included the voices and perspectives of people with dementia?

- Showing the potential hope in stories of life with dementia is a radical act, and it sits against an abundance of stories of despair. How will your story balance the ups and downs of life with dementia in a way that creates community rather than fear?

Acknowledgements

We would like to thank everyone who was part of creating *Maggie May* for their tremendous creativity, courage and care.

Leeds Playhouse is a major producing theatre with a reputation for socially engaged practice with communities and world-class stage productions.

References

Basting, A. D. (1998) *The Stages of Age: Performing Age in Contemporary American Culture.* Ann Arbor, MI: University of Michigan Press.

Basting, A. (2006) 'Beyond the stigma of Alzheimer's.' *Journal of Medical Humanities 27*, 125–126.

Chansky, D. (2023) 'Inside (and) Out: "Who Exactly Am I?"—*The Father.*' In: *Losing It.* Cham: Palgrave Macmillan.

Escolme, B. (2018) 'When grief has mates: King Lear and the politics of happiness.' *The Lancet, Psychiatry 5*, 8, 621–622.

Taylor, P. and Poet, F. (2020) 'How Maggie May Came to Life – Reflections on the Process.' In F. Poet (2020) *Maggie May.* London: Nick Hern Books.

Tuijt, R., Frost, R., Wilcock, J., Robinson, L. *et al.* (2021) 'Life under lockdown and social restrictions: The experiences of people living with dementia and their carers during the COVID-19 pandemic in England.' *B BMC Geriatrics 21*, 1, 301.

Zeilig, H. (2012) 'Dementia as cultural metaphor.' *The Gerontologist 54*, 2, 258–267.

CHAPTER 8

House of Memories

Carol Rogers

Introduction

Carol Rogers was head of learning at National Museums Liverpool (NML) when a family experience of dementia prompted her to explore how museums could use their collections to develop resources that trigger memories for people living with dementia, share these memories with formal and informal carers and play a more active role in raising awareness of dementia.

This chapter sets the development of the House of Memories (HoM) programme in the context of the modernisation of UK museums. It highlights the critical role of NML and its support for the pioneering co-created HoM programme and My House of Memories app, which stimulate memories of people living with dementia and their carers. The case example describes the co-production of a culturally appropriate Yemeni community HoM programme, including a culturally relevant app, whilst the expansion of the HoM programme nationally and internationally attests to the value of the resource for museums and dementia communities worldwide.

The UK museum sector

For decades, traditional museums collected, preserved and displayed objects for public education, albeit this presented an exclusive view of art, culture and history, largely reflecting the prestige and privilege of small and self-selected groups of visitors. From the 1990s, however, socio-economic change, including a challenging funding environment, remodelled museums' roles, functions and activities. Museums began to grow and diversify audiences and widen access. Passive cultural consumption was largely replaced by active participation, and digitalisation of museum collections increased opportunities for interaction. When national and local government policies shifted to place-making and localism, local agencies and museum partnerships were established to engage communities in health and wellbeing improvement and foster social inclusion.

Lockdown during the COVID-19 pandemic accelerated these trends. Most museums have now hybridised their offer, so alongside in-person visits, the museum *experience* of learning and entertainment, and increasingly, a personalised experience, are provided through digital, virtual and augmented technologies including apps, projection mapping, and AI.

National Museums Liverpool

National Museums Liverpool (NML) is a group of seven world-leading museums and galleries, located across Liverpool City Region. The group's museums and galleries host an encyclopaedic collection of more than 4 million objects, ranging from some of the world's best Pre-Raphaelite artworks to an awe-inspiring Ancient Egypt collection, and more recently, the UK's only modern slavery museum collection.

The core mission and focus of NML is to educate, enable unheard perspectives to be voiced, support social change, and inspire and connect with people of all ages and diversity, in person and online. NML has supported the development of HoM – a unique museum education programme and resources that support dementia communities worldwide.

The development of the House of Memories programme

The impetus for the development of HoM was the recognition that museums are keepers of memories and that NML and other UK museums have a wealth of local historical and socio-cultural objects, photographs and documents that can be used to prompt memories of people living with dementia.

Unusually for a museum, NML took a direct interest in supporting the HoM team, who embarked on developing a memory programme co-created with people living with dementia and their carers as active participants in the production process and in generating a museum-based digital narrative. The HoM team learnt about communicating effectively with people with dementia, including writing for people living with dementia (Innovations in Dementia 2013), and enabled participants to positively engage with the development, design and piloting of a digital resource – an app that can be personalised.

The HoM team collaborated with Mersey Care Hospital Trust, a provider of acute care for people living with dementia, and Liverpool John Moores

University. The university's Living Lab was used in the development of HoM to ensure that users, as co-creators, were at the centre of the research-to-innovation-to-solution process, the ethos of co-creation with people with dementia was rigorously applied throughout the work and the innovation met the needs and requirements of the dementia community.

The co-creation process is informed by an established Integrated Knowledge Transfer (IKT) approach whereby people living with dementia are designated 'knowledge users' and supported as shared partners throughout the co-development of the intervention/product/service to its proposed delivery. This follows a four-stage process: start-up/planning, content development, intervention and protocol (Smith *et al.* 2022).

The process of all HoM programme development is underpinned by real-world co-creation and representation. Each programme is externally evaluated, providing the HoM team with learning and tools that are disseminated to the wider museum sector.

Since 2012, this successful programme has expanded its range of activities and projects to include the following areas of work:

Dementia training

The original programme was primarily designed to deliver a training programme for the UK social care sector about using a 'dementia education' weblink to information about museum objects and social history collections. These resources can be used to support person-centred approaches to dementia care by facilitating personal memories and triggering socially and culturally rich memories about family lives and community identities.

The programme soon evolved into a larger, more diverse resource. UK place-based museum training events were run supported by a range of multi-language supplementary resources, including the My House of Memories app, a digital memory resource for iPads and other tablets.

My House of Memories app

Individuals living with dementia and their carers can use a digital device such as a smartphone or iPad to access and save data about NML objects and images. These can be used to create a personalised viewable digital memory experience that can be shared with others. Access and digital inclusion for older users was promoted by Connect My Memories, an app loan service including a training workshop with support from an online facilitator.

Downloading the app facilitates access to a wide range of UK, USA and Singaporean social history content linked to stories and objects from 1920 to

1980, accompanied by music and film designed to prompt discussion between users about everyday memories and events, for example, school life, sport, food or transport. Selected objects can be saved to a digital memory tree or personal memory album to share with friends and family.

For older people and those living with dementia, the app provides a unique way to digitise and share their memories with families, neighbours and community networks. Retrieving memories can reinforce a sense of identity and belonging. However, people living with dementia, especially as they become more cognitively impaired, experience difficulties in perception of past and present time (time-shifting). Getting to know individuals and/or involving family carers or care staff in creating a digitalised memory experience can reduce the risks of triggering anxiety by including less well remembered objects or events or those often associated with loss and trauma such as war.

House of Memories activities: On the Road

In order to engage with older people and communities least served by the museum sector, HOM staff have developed a wide range of projects, diverse in locality and reach. Regular activities in Liverpool include monthly memory walks at the Museum of Liverpool and community digital outreach training sessions.

In 2021, the HoM team developed On the Road, an immersive mobile museum experience for older people, including those living with dementia, that is designed as an interactive cinema experience that stimulates conversations about shared local histories and memories. A community vehicle travels to Liverpool neighbourhoods, and audience members sit in comfort and immerse themselves in 3D films of local streets, shops and trips to the seaside, accompanied by sound, images and smells that evoke memories of past times. The aim is simple: when you can't get to the museum, the museum comes to you.

The HoM programme offers a model of evidence-based person-centred dementia practice and resources for people living with dementia that can be used by all types and size of museum with multiple and diverse collections. There are a wealth of different HoM resources available at www.liverpool-museums.org.uk/house-of-memories.

Programme case study: Connecting with Yemeni Elders Heritage

HoM was designed to enable people living with dementia and their carers to elicit and share knowledge and understanding about an individual's life history and life experience. The HOM team acknowledged that the

Western historical and cultural resources providing source content for the My House of Memories app were unlikely to stimulate memories for an individual from a different ethnic and socio-cultural background, and this was confirmed in 2021 when Abdul Wase, a young person from Liverpool's Yemeni community, having discovered the My House of Memories app, approached the HOM team seeking culturally appropriate resources to support the care of his grandmother who is living with dementia.

In response to Abdul's request for an app with Yemeni cultural heritage content, the HoM team began to scope out the intergenerational Connecting with Yemeni Elders Heritage project with Abdul and a group of his peers, the Liverpool Kuumba Imani Millennium Centre, Liverpool Arabic Centre, Liverpool Arabic Arts Festival, the Al-Ghazali Centre, Al-Taiseer Mosque and The Studio School. Liverpool John Moores University was commissioned to evaluate the project (Wilson 2022).

Managed by a Connecting with Yemeni Elders Heritage steering group, the project had three outcomes – to:

- co-create an intergenerational programme that facilitated engagement with Yemeni elders and young people and increased cultural awareness and understanding of access to collections
- showcase the objects and stories of a Liverpool Yemeni community and museum collections within the framework of the My House of Memories app to connect and support the community's ageing population, including those members living with dementia
- support the UK museum sector in developing a model for collaborating with young people to create community collections that align, connect and interpret museum collections.

The project was delivered over two years. In the first year, a community project leader was recruited from the Liverpool Yemeni community to support a project advisory group, created in consultation with stakeholders. Together, they led on the development of the co-production workshops to explore museum collections, community objects and stories. Partner museum collections and public digital collections were also accessed to develop new stories and include additional object references.

The team was supported by a group of Yemeni young people, who led the intergenerational co-curation work with the HoM team. Their contributions varied from giving speeches and talking to the media, to volunteering at events and recording the app object narrative.

In the second year, the intergenerational group conducted community testing, gathered feedback, agreed final digital content, signed off presentations and produced a guide and toolkit for young people and interested museums. More information can be found at:

- https://youtu.be/poaSxE3fbSw
- www.liverpoolmuseums.org.uk/house-of-memories/my-house-of-memories-app
- www.liverpoolmuseums.org.uk/house-of-memories/toolkit

Connecting with Yemeni Elders
Heritage project: learning points

The project facilitated learning about developing a partnership between a museum, a marginalised local community and local partners. Key learning points, which were shared with UK museums, are summarised below:

Community engagement: It is important to establish community connections and clear communication and relationships with your stakeholders and community leaders prior to exploring the potential of working together, co-design, project initiation and co-development. Allocating sufficient time to building community relationships and getting to know the area is crucial. Attending networking events can help museum staff familiarise themselves with the community's cultural heritage and identify possible connections to museum collections and venue settings.

Project development: A shared project delivery framework needs to be developed in consultation with key community representatives, together with nominating a link person, either from your team or a community-based project coordinator (budget permitting). A programme schedule for project development, including content co-production and progress reporting plus an overview of the budget (where appropriate), needs to be agreed. Any information communicated about collaboration and co-production needs to be in plain English, limiting 'museum speak', as jargon can unintentionally alienate stakeholders. An evaluation framework for internal assessment and external sharing needs to be agreed, together with an external research partner (academic) to carry out the evaluation.

Project delivery: Setting up a community steering group with stakeholder representation can help identify community settings and assets that relate to and connect with your project. Support ongoing engagement through sharing regular project updates at community events, and participate in cultural celebrations and anniversaries. Ensure a regular project newsletter is produced and circulated amongst all project members.

Project legacy: Celebrate project progress and achievement in your museum and with community partners in local settings. Key outputs include a documentary film of the project's development and delivery to share with advocates and stakeholders through social media and news outlets, and a public record of learning outcomes. Build on success and explore the potential to replicate your approach with other community groups.

Working at scale: To sustain, share and develop your learning, explore the potential to expand your project with multiple museum partners and communities by developing a replicable project delivery methodology for new partners and designing a structure that can be delivered within different museum settings (city and rural) with different partners (volunteer, local authority and national museums). Distributing your project impact evaluation to interested partners and producing a strategy to promote and celebrate your achievements maintains the high profile of your work.

House of Memories: development and expansion

One of the more ambitious aims of the NML development of HoM was to encourage museums across the world to tailor the content of the My House of Memories app and use it to support their local dementia communities. Over the last decade, the programme has reached more than 100,000 people, and there have been 38,000 downloads of the My House of Memories app. Multi-language digital resources were developed in Arabic, Chinese Mandarin, Tamil and Malay. The HoM team has continued to diversify and expand the programme through:

- House of Memories Cymru, a bilingual model co-produced with 14 museum partners across Wales
- a football memories resource with Liverpool Football Club Foundation
- a digital package for UK veterans
- a digital package for the LGBTQ+ dementia community.

The HoM team hopes to explore further global partnerships with museums in Southeast Asia, the USA and South America.

Conclusion

In the 1990s, the roles and functions of UK museums began to change; NML championed many of these changes in widening access to its collections, promoting social inclusion and cultural diversity, and acting as a focal point for its local community through building partnerships. This milieu was supportive of developing a museum-based community engagement programme that responded to the needs of people living with dementia and their informal and formal carers.

The HoM programme was co-created by NML with people living with dementia and their carers, Mersey Care Hospital Trust and Liverpool John Moores University. Objects, photographs and other material from social and cultural heritage collections held by NML and UK museums were used to develop training, digital content for the My House of Memories app and outreach activities and projects. The HoM team worked in partnership with members of Liverpool's Yemeni community and local agencies to produce Connecting with Yemeni Elders Heritage, a culturally appropriate HoM programme for older people, including those living with dementia.

The HoM programme enables people living with dementia to access and enjoy museum collections that serve to trigger memories. In doing so, it delivers on key principles of best practice in creative arts and dementia – diversity, equity, inclusion – that museums strive to offer worldwide. Small wonder, then, that HoM has been adopted globally and is changing care through arts and culture.

LEARNING POINTS

The HoM programme provides a case study of how a national museum (NML) has gone beyond the traditional museum visiting experience by using its collection for a social purpose. It is important to note the following points:

- NML's support for a dedicated in-house team. The museum recognised the need to resource a partnership approach that involved extensive co-design and co-production of the HoM programme with people living with dementia, family carers, Mersey Care Hospital Trust and Liverpool John Moores University.

- The value of working with a specialist app company. The HoM programme combined artistic interpretation, curatorship, museum education and reminiscence therapy techniques in developing an app that triggers memories through museum objects, artefacts, images, etc.

- The HoM learning programme designed to raise awareness of dementia and how to use the app in working with individuals with the condition can be accessed by families and health and social care professionals in several ways, including online and face to face.

- Dissemination of the app and learning programme: the HoM app can be customised to deliver specific memory content and in different languages as exemplified in the local Yemeni Elders Heritage project community and its use with other community groups, other UK museums and other countries.

References

Innovations in Dementia (2013) Deep guide: Writing dementia friendly information. http://dementiavoices.org.uk/wp-content/uploads/2013/11/DEEP-Guide-Writing-dementia-friendly-information.pdf

Smith, G., Dixon, C., Ganga, R. and Greenop, D. (2022) 'How do we know co-created solutions work effectively within the real world of people living with dementia? Learning methodological lessons from a co-creation-to-evaluation case study.' *International Journal of Environmental Research and Public Health* 19, 21.

Wilson, J. (2022) Connecting with Yemeni Elders Heritage. National Museums, Liverpool. www.liverpoolmuseums.org.uk/house-of-memories/connecting-yemeni-elders-heritage

CHAPTER 9

Creative Arts in Care Homes

Maria Pasiecznik Parsons, Alison Teader
and Hilary Woodhead

This chapter contextualises the needs of care home residents living with dementia and how these are met by Activity Providers, who organise and provide activities in conjunction with staff. Some care providers and care homes commission experienced creative arts practitioners, but there are many that experience barriers to doing so. The National Activity Providers Association (NAPA) and the Baring Foundation provide resources for managers, and staff can help them to promote partnership working between care providers, care homes, arts organisations and local communities. These foster creative communities and facilitate creativity in care homes, but making creativity and culture regularly available for residents in all care homes requires a wider systems approach.

Care homes: person-centred care for an active life

Some 70% of people living in UK care homes have dementia and, of these, over half have severe dementia activities (Cutler 2022). In England, care homes are regulated, registered and inspected by the Care Quality Commission (CQC), an independent non-departmental government body. There are separate regulatory bodies for Wales, Scotland and Northern Ireland. A care home can be registered as a residential or nursing home; people living with dementia may live in both types of home, but those with complex care needs are more likely to live in nursing homes that provide nursing care.

All care homes have a legal duty to provide safe person-centred care that supports personal development, social activity and wellbeing. Additionally, the National Institute for Health and Care Excellence (NICE) guideline QS50 stipulates that 'meaningful activity should be provided in care homes and that residents should be provided with support to engage in activities in line with their abilities and preferences' (NICE 2013).

After admission, a new resident will be allocated a key worker, usually a care assistant, who will spend time talking to them about their life history, including where they were born and grew up, family histories, education, employment, interests and hobbies. Relatives or friends may be involved and can help fill in any gaps. The key worker combines biographical information and information about the resident's physical and cognitive health to assess their strengths and needs and then develops a care plan that optimises a resident's independence and supports their care choices. Details are recorded in a full care plan, whilst a shorter daily care plan is used by staff on duty to help them meet a resident's daily living needs, including how they like to spend their day. The care plan is monitored, regularly reviewed and updated with the resident, their family or friends.

Activities, Activity Providers and creative arts

Care home residents living with dementia are more likely to have unmet social needs, particularly for company and daytime activities (Hancock *et al.* 2005) that result in boredom, loneliness and under-occupation (Smit *et al.* 2016), all of which can exacerbate psychological and behavioural symptoms of dementia (Ferreira, Dias and Fernande 2016). Compared with residents living with dementia whose time was unstructured, Cohen-Mansfield (2018) found that individuals who participated in structured group activities, for example, games and choral singing, demonstrated improvements in engagement, cognition and behaviour, and that these were greater for residents with moderate to severe dementia. Ensuring care home residents are regularly involved in activities that are 'co-produced' (Robertson and McCall, 2018) and meaningful to individuals and tailored to their interests, hobbies and cultural choices and preferences contributes to their quality of life (Smit *et al.* 2016, Tierney *et al.* 2023).

Most homes employ an Activities Provider, sometimes known as an Activities Organiser or a Lifestyle Lead (larger homes may employ more), to organise activities to meet residents' needs, especially their physical, psychological and social needs. Besides working with groups, Activity Providers also provide one-to-one support for residents with behavioural and cognitive symptoms of dementia or with complex physical care needs, including residents who are bedfast and those receiving palliative care.

There are an estimated 8000 Activity Providers working in UK care homes, of whom 1800 (22.5%) are NAPA-accredited Activity Professionals. Their rewarding roles are not without challenges: whilst almost half feel supported in their work, many have unmet training and professional development needs, below industry average salary levels and high workloads (NAPA 2024).

Hence, it is important that Activity Providers work with an experienced, stable, trained staff group who use person-centred care, which is strongly associated with care home quality (Spilsbury *et al.* 2024). Currently, only 45% of care home staff receive dementia care training and few learn about working creatively, yet training staff in person-centred care and social interaction using the Wellbeing and Health for People Living with Dementia (WHELD) programme improved residents' quality of life, reduced levels of agitation and antipsychotic use, and cost less to deliver than usual care (Ballard *et al.* 2018).

Creative arts practitioners in care homes

A whole-home approach to creativity includes management, leadership and staff support for Activity Providers. Research shows that residents benefit from creative arts provided by experienced practitioners. These benefits include reciprocal social relationships, belongingness and social cohesion (Dadswell *et al.* 2020) and a sense of purpose and resilience in residents (Newman *et al.* 2019), whilst music positively affects the cognition and attention of people living with dementia and boosts self-identity and self-esteem (McDermott, Orrell and Ridder 2014).

Besides fostering inclusion, integration and a sense of identity, Tapson *et al.* (2018) found that joint working with musicians changed staff views about the value of music for residents. This chimes with a study by Lawrence *et al.* (2013), who found that involvement in creative arts can help overcome staff scepticism about the value of non-pharmacological care approaches and that 'merely participating in psychosocial interventions, such as life-review work or music events, helped staff to see beyond the symptoms of dementia and to broaden their conceptualisation of the caregiving role' (*ibid.* p.48).

Staff participation in creative arts sessions improved their understanding of residents' strengths and needs and the value of non-verbal communication besides giving them confidence to try more creative approaches to care (Windle *et al.* 2020). These findings resonate with results of the cARTrefu project in Wales that evidenced the social value of creative arts; participating staff were also more likely to engage in cultural activities (i.e. arts classes, visiting gallery/theatre) outside of work (Algar-Skaife, Caulfield and Woods 2017).

Staff participants often discover new biographical information about residents and their interests, enabling them to better tailor and support a resident's creativity and gain confidence in applying creativity to care routines

(Broome *et al.* 2017). In one Central and Cecil care home, Alison Teader, former Project Manager of Arts in Care Homes in Central and Cecil Housing Trust recalls that:

> …staff sang to relax anxious residents living with dementia whilst taking them to the toilet or hoisting them out of chairs. Residents reluctant to enter the dining room for meals were encouraged to do so by a staff member who danced alongside them whilst another used playful drama games with a lady who loved horses: galloping and swishing 'tails' with much shared hilarity.

Barriers to creative arts in care homes

Residents' access to creativity and cultural activity in UK care homes is a lottery of provision. Research Scotland (2022) found that barriers include lack of expertise or confidence to commission structured creative arts sessions amongst care providers, whilst managers' lack of specialist knowledge of creative engagement for residents inhibits them from commissioning experienced creative arts practitioners. *A Manager's Guide to Arts in Care Homes* (NAPA 2023) provides resources, support, guidance and tools for managers seeking to develop creative, connected, vibrant communities in care homes, helping a manager to lead by example and model a rights-based approach to enabling residents to live creative and fulfilled lives.

Smit *et al.* (2016) found that activating and supporting residents required flexing staff duties and reducing instrumental work demands, improving education levels and ensuring all staff are trained to use activities during daily care. Many of these findings resonate with the results of a NAPA survey that sought answers to the question of 'What would it require for all care homes to offer their residents access to relevant creative and cultural opportunities on a daily basis?' Staff wanted (more) resources, dedicated time, creative ideas, community partnerships, access to digital devices and resources, training and teamwork; residents identified a range of creative arts and opportunities that they would welcome; relatives, having noted the benefits of arts and culture, wanted there to be a daily offer and to be able to join in (Cutler 2022).

Nevertheless, costs are a major deterrent for many care providers. A mapping of creative activities in Scottish care settings including care homes (Stevenson 2018) highlights costs as a major consideration, since care homes may have to double-fund sessions: paying the fees of creative arts practitioners and back-filling (covering staff) staff involved, sometimes by hiring agency staff. Larger providers such as C&C have advantages of scale, staff capacity, a dedicated central budget for creative arts provision and capacity to collaborate with arts and cultural organisations to apply for and secure local and national funding, for example, from The National Lottery or charitable trusts. They are also more likely to host longer residencies led by established arts organisations, such as Magic Me, Music in Mind, Living Words and Green Candle Dance, and to have sufficient staff resources and minibuses to be able to access dementia-friendly programmes in museums, galleries, theatres and cinemas. Smaller care home providers often commission local freelance creative arts practitioners for sessional work. Many providers hold fundraising events to generate funds and/or ask relatives and friends to donate materials. Volunteers, including minibus drivers, are an invaluable resource.

Better together: care homes and arts organisations working together

Improving standards of care is a strong driver for arts and care partnerships. CQC (2016) defines an outstanding service as one that is 'flexible and responsive to people's individual needs and preferences, finding creative ways to enable people to live a full life.' According to Live Music Now, a high proportion of English care homes rated as outstanding offer dedicated music for residents (Tapson *et al.* 2018). Some organisations provide in-house creative arts, including Methodist Homes (MHA) care homes, whose 22 music therapists offer music therapy to 22,000 residents across 65 of its 83 care homes. Community Integrated Care has a partnership with Age Exchange to provide creative arts in their care homes.

Such collaboration and partnership between creative arts practitioners, arts organisations and care providers results in high-quality arts provision (Bungay *et al.* 2021), enabling them to overcome many of the barriers that providers experience in enabling residents to access creative arts and cultural activities (Cutler 2022). Models of good practice include:

- cARTrefu, a long-running national creative arts in care homes programme in Wales, was established and supported by the Arts Council of Wales, Age Cymru, Gwanwyn and the Baring Foundation (Algar-Skaife *et al.* 2017).

- Dare to Imagine, an Artists' Residencies in Care Homes (ARCH) programme, 2019–2023, was developed and run by a collaboration between Magic Me, artistic partners and Excelcare homes. Key outputs include the final project report (Wilson *et al.*, 2023) and a guide to care home activities (Magic Me 2024).

- Arts in Care Homes (AICH) is an annual NAPA programme that aims to highlight the health and wellbeing benefits of arts, creativity and cultural engagement in care settings. Culminating in a National Arts in Care Homes Day in the UK and internationally, it involves many thousands of care home residents, families, staff and arts health and community organisations showcasing creative activities that contribute to quality of life in care homes.

Music for Life: an arts and care homes partnership project

There were many positive outcomes for residents and staff who participated in an arts and social care partnership between C&C and Music for Life. Typically, professional musicians started with sessions around rhythm, using percussion instruments and clapping exercises.

Alison Teader, former Project Manager of Arts in Care Homes in Central and Cecil Housing Trust noted the following:

It was fascinating to see how the participating people living with dementia retained their sense of rhythm and recall of song words. Staff joined in the sessions and the project brought great happiness into the care home and seemed to contribute to feelings of belongingness and community. One participant, a woman in her late 80s, told us she couldn't join in a singing session as her teacher had told her she 'growled like a bear', and as a result, she had not sung since. The musicians persevered, inviting her to join us every week. At the end of the last session, after she had finally joined in, we heard her saying excitedly to a member of care staff, 'Did you hear me? I can sing!'

Care homes and creative connections

The COVID-19 pandemic highlighted the interdependencies between care homes and local communities, showing how:

...much of the resilience in the system was a consequence of dedicated and resourceful staff using existing local networks, or forging new ones, to work around the challenges brought forward both by the pandemic and the central policy decisions intended to deal with it. (Marshall, Gordon and Gladman 2021)

Staff played key roles in supporting residents to remain active during lockdowns using hands-on and online arts resources (Cutler 2020). Both staff and residents gained confidence in using smartphones and tablets, and the digitalisation of online arts and cultural resources (Misek, Leguina and Man-ninen 2022) widened inclusion and increased their access to museum collec-tions as well as to online art, music, dance and poetry sessions uploaded by creative arts practitioners. NAPA brokered a partnership with the University of Exeter that enabled care home residents and staff to engage in Culture Box, a project that offered physical and digital arts materials, visual arts, music and nature-based activities (Tischler *et al.* 2023).

NAPA and Innovations in Dementia set up and supported an online Dementia Craftivists project that connected care home residents, Activity Providers and staff to community-dwelling people living with experience and/or interest in arts. This group ran online sessions offering different arts activities for small groups of residents and staff.

Gallistl, Seifert and Kolland (2021), however, concluded that care homes might find staff commitment to embedding and maintaining online arts par-ticipation – particularly regular digital engagement and hybrid participation, together with ongoing training and learning – hard to sustain.

Creative communities

Care homes can be envisaged as 'creative communities' – places where resi-dents, including people living with dementia, enjoy: being creative together, alongside staff, relatives, friends and volunteers; learning new skills, sharing learning and expertise; and having the chance to be creative in a variety of person-centred ways through access to different art forms. Some care homes have cafe areas and other communal spaces that staff use to provide oppor-tunities for people in the local community to join in activities and share their skills with residents, families and local groups, besides welcoming them in for film nights and other events.

As the Dementia Craftivists project demonstrated, digital access also enables care homes to make links with community resources via apps includ-ing Armchair Gallery (City Arts Nottingham) and the House of Memories (National Museums Liverpool, see Chapter 8). Virtual reality (VR), such as The Wayback project, enables residents living with dementia to reminisce as they virtually experience Queen Elizabeth II Coronation street parties (The Wayback 2024).

Many Activity Providers and staff nurture their connections with local communities, including arts, cultural and heritage venues that over the past 20 years have become more dementia friendly (Allen *et al.* 2015), offering people living with dementia, including those in care homes, opportunities to participate in specially curated programmes such as Sensory Palaces offered by Historic Royal Palaces and health and wellbeing activities at Beamish Museum.

Many venues have developed customised resources such as boxes of objects, ephemera and photographs that can be handled by residents during reminiscence sessions. These range from coinage reminiscence boxes produced by the Royal Mint Museum, South Wales to the Museum of Cornish Life loan boxes designed to help care home residents recall aspects of local life and language.

Bristol Care Homes run intergenerational programmes in partnership with Alive Activities and local schools using arts, music and horticultural activities to enhance understanding between the generations and reduce stereotypes and stigma. In partnership with three care homes, The Alzheimer's Society (2025) has produced a care home community engagement toolkit to encourage care homes to become catalysts for community engagement whereby residents and staff benefit from increased social connections whilst helping to build local social capital.

Huge potential exists for 'every care home [to become] a creative home' but, as Cutler (2022) argues, a systems approach is required across arts and social care and needs to include the government, care homes, the CQC, care home infrastructure bodies, arts organisations and artists, and arts funders, including Arts Council England.

Conclusion: creative lives for care home residents living with dementia

Evidence underpins mandatory guidance to care homes about the value of meaningful person-centred activities and creative arts for care home residents living with dementia. In most homes, an Activity Provider organises and leads a weekly and annual schedule of activities to meet the physical, psychological and social needs of a diverse (and often large) group. Almost 25% of Activity Providers have completed NAPA training for what is a rewarding but challenging role for which manager and staff support is vital.

Adopting a whole-home approach to creativity includes commissioning creative arts led by experienced practitioners who can deliver a range of specific benefits for residents. Managers can play a key role in facilitating the provision of creative arts in care homes that benefits residents, relatives and staff.

Barriers to commissioning and using external creative arts practitioners include care providers' knowledge of creative arts, staff capacity and costs, particularly for smaller providers. Many of these barriers can be overcome by building partnerships with local communities, schools, and arts and heritage organisations, as well as by accessing online resources for enabling care homes to become creative communities, whilst the goal of a daily offer of creativity in care homes requires a wider systems approach.

LEARNING POINTS

Outcomes for residents in care homes are enhanced when:

- creative arts and activities are personalised

- experienced and trained Activity Providers work with staff, families and volunteers to plan and organise opportunities for activities, creative arts and cultural engagement

- care providers support managers who commission creative arts practitioners to work with Activity Providers and upskill staff

- care homes are an integral part of the local community

- care providers and arts organisations work in partnership to develop and deliver sustainable creative arts programmes.

All NAPA resources can be accessed at https://napa-activities.co.uk, and publications about creativity in care homes can be downloaded at https://baring-foundation.org.uk.

References

Algar-Skaife, K., Caulfield, M. and Woods, B. (2017) *cARTrefu: Creating Artists in Residents. A National Arts in Care Homes Participatory and Mentoring Programme. Evaluation report 2015–2017.* Bangor: DSDC Wales Report, Bangor University, School of Healthcare Sciences.

Allen, P., Brown, A., Camic, P.M., Cutler, D., *et al.* (2015) *Dementia Friendly Arts Venues.* London: Alzheimer's Society. www.alzheimers.org.uk/sites/default/files/2019-07/AS_DF_NEW_Arts_Guide_Online_09_07_19.pdf

Alzheimer's Society (2025) The care home and community engagement toolkit. www.alzheimers.org.uk/get-involved/dementia-friendly-communities/care-home-community-engagement-toolkit

Ballard, C., Corbett, A., Orrell, M., Williams, G., *et al.* (2018) 'Impact of person-centred care training and person-centred activities on quality of life, agitation, and antipsychotic use in people with dementia living in nursing homes: A cluster-randomised controlled trial.' *PLOS Medicine 15, 2, e1002500.*

Broome, E., Dening, T., Schneider, J. and Brooker, D. (2017) 'Care staff and the creative arts: exploring the context of involving care personnel in arts interventions.' *International Psychogeriatrics 29, 1979–1991.*

Bungay, H., Wilson, C., Dadswell A. and Munn-Giddings, C. (2021) 'The role of collaborative working between arts and care sectors in successfully delivering participatory arts activities for older people in residential care settings.' *Health and Social Care in the Community* 29, 6, 1807–1814.

Care Quality Commission (2016) *The Art of Being Outstanding.* Presentation by Andrea Sutcliffe, Chief Inspector, Care Quality Commission. https://carequalitycomm.medium.com/the-art-of-being-outstanding-86c21a9449c3

Cohen-Mansfield, J. (2018) 'The impact of group activities and their content on persons with dementia attending them.' *Alzheimer's Research and Therapy* 10, 37.

Cutler, D. (2020) *Key Workers Creative Ageing in Lockdown and After.* London: The Baring Foundation. https://cdn.baringfoundation.org.uk/wp-content/uploads/BF_Key-workers_WEB_lr-1.pdf

Cutler, D. (2022) *Every Care Home a Creative Home: A Systems Approach to Personalised Creativity and Culture.* London: The Baring Foundation. https://cdn.baringfoundation.org.uk/wp-content/uploads/BF_Every-care-home_FINAL.pdf

Dadswell, A., Bungay, H., Wilson, C. and Munn-Giddings, C. (2020) 'The impact of participatory arts in promoting social relationships for older people within care homes.' *Perspectives in Public Health* 140, 5, 286–293.

Dementia Creatives (2021) Connecting with people living in care homes through Craftivism. https://dementiacreatives.org.uk/craftnewsitems/connecting-with-people-living-in-care-homes-through-craftivism

Ferreira, A. R, Dias, C. C. and Fernandes, L. (2016) 'Needs in nursing homes and their relation with cognitive and functional decline, behavioral and psychological symptoms.' *Frontiers in Aging Neuroscience* 8, 1–10.

Gallistl, V., Seifert, A. and Kolland, F. (2021) 'COVID-19 as a "digital push?" Research experiences from long-term care and recommendations for the post-pandemic era.' *Frontiers in Public Health* 9, 660064.

Hancock, G, A., Woods, R., Challis D. and Orrell, M. (2005) 'The needs of older people with dementia in residential care.' *International Journal of Geriatric Psychiatry* 21, 43–49.

Lawrence, V., Fossey, J., Ballard, C., Moniz-Cook, E. and Murray, J. (2013) 'Improving quality of life for people with dementia in care homes: Making psychosocial interventions work.' *British Journal of Psychiatry* 201, 5, 344–351.

Magic Me (2024) *A Care Home's Guide to Creativity.* London: Magic Me. https://magicme.co.uk/wp-content/uploads/2024/02/Dare-to-Imagine-a-care-homes-guide-to-creativity.pdf

Marshall, F., Gordon, A. and Gladman, J. (2021) 'Care homes, their communities, and resilience in the face of the COVID-19 pandemic: Interim findings from a qualitative study.' *BMC Geriatics* 21, 1, 102.

McDermott, O., Orrell, M. and Ridder, H. M. (2014) 'The importance of music for people with dementia: The perspectives of people with dementia, family carers, staff and music therapists.' *Aging Mental Health* 18, 6, 706–716.

Misek, R., Leguina, A. and Manninen, K. (2022) *Digital Access to Arts and Culture.* Loughborough: Loughborough University. https://hdl.handle.net/2134/20025731.v1

NAPA (2023) *A Manager's Guide to Arts in Care Homes.* London: NAPA and The Baring Foundation. https://cdn.baringfoundation.org.uk/wp-content/uploads/Care-home-managers-NAPA-2023.pdf

NAPA (2024) *National Activity Provider Survey Analysis Summary.* https://digital.napa-activities.co.uk/view/829344240

National Institute for Health and Care Excellence (2013) *Mental Wellbeing of Older People in Care Homes. Quality Standard* (QS50). www.nice.org.uk/guidance/qs50

Newman, A., Goulding, A., Davenport, B. and Windle, G. (2019) 'The role of the visual arts in the resilience of people living with dementia in care homes.' *Ageing and Society* 39, 11, 2465–2482.

Research Scotland (2022) *Evaluation of the Arts in Care Project.* https://luminatescotland.org/wp-content/uploads/2023/03/Arts-in-Care-Final-Report-January-2023.pdf

Robertson, J. M. and McCall, V. (2018) 'Facilitating creativity in dementia care: The co-construction of arts-based engagement.' *Ageing and Society* 40, 6, 1155–1174.

Smit, D., De Lange, J., Willemse, B., Twisk, J. and Pot, A. M. (2016) 'Activity involvement and quality of life of people at different stages of dementia in long term care facilities.' *Aging & Mental Health* 20, 1, 100–109.

Spilsbury, K., Charlwood, A., Thompson, C., Haunch, K. *et al.* (2024) 'Relationship between staff and quality of care in care homes: StaRQ mixed methods study.' *Health and Social Care Delivery Research* 12, 8.

Stevenson, R. (2018) *Final Report for Luminate, Scotland, Mapping of Creative Activities in Scottish Care Settings.* Edinburgh: Ruthless Research.

Tapson, C., Noble, D., Daykin, N. and Walters, D. (2018) *Live Music in Care: The Impact of Music Interventions for People Living and Working in Care Homes for Residents in Care Homes.* Winchester: University of Winchester. https://achoirineverycarehome.files.wordpress.com/2018/11/live-music-in-care.pdf

The Wayback (2024) The Wayback homepage. https://thewaybackvr.com

Tierney, L., MacAndrew, M., Doherty, K., Fielding, E. and Beattie, E. (2023) 'Characteristics and value of "meaningful activity" for people living with dementia in residential aged care facilities: "You're still part of the world, not just existing".' *Dementia, International Journal of Social Research and Practice* 22, 2.

Tischler, V., Zeilig, H., O'Malley, M. and Asker, C. (2023) 'Together yet apart: Rethinking creativity and relational dementia care during the Covid-19 pandemic.' *Geriatric Nursing* 54, 99–107.

Wilson, C., Dadswell, A., Bungay, H. and Munn-Giddins, C. (2023) *Dare to Imagine: Artists and Care Home Staff Working Together to Embed Creativity in Care Homes. Artists' Residencies in Care Homes Programme 2019–23.* Magic Me and Anglia Ruskin University. https://flipbooks.gs-cdn.co.uk/aru-magic-me

Windle, G., Algar-Skaife, K., Caulfield, M., Pickering-Jones, L. *et al.* (2020) 'Enhancing communication between dementia care staff and their residents: An arts-inspired intervention.' *Aging & Mental Health* 24, 8, 1306–1315.

CHAPTER 10

Creative Arts in Hospitals

Angela Conlan, Paula Har, Richard Coaten
and Maria Pasiecznik Parsons

Introduction

Imagine that you are stepping into a bustling hospital ward filled with the sounds of beeping machines, hurried footsteps and hushed conversations. When you do this, you are also stepping into a ward culture that is a unique blend of professionalism, compassion and multidisciplinary teamwork. Staff dart from one patient to another, diligently attending to their needs whilst aiming to maintain a calm and organised environment.

Creative Practitioners in hospitals are working in unique settings and would therefore benefit from understanding aspects of a very complex system of care and treatment, particularly about effective joint working with a multidisciplinary hospital ward team. This can help them to navigate challenges and personalise approaches, particularly in respect of the behavioural and physiological symptoms of dementia, as well as identifying who might benefit from a non-pharmacological approach like drawing, music or poetry.

This chapter provides good practice guidance for creative arts practitioners who work or wish to work in hospital settings by describing:

- the hospital experience of older patients, especially those living with dementia, and their needs
- the benefits of arts in hospitals
- arts teams in hospitals
- good practice in hospital arts
- arts for staff wellbeing
- arts and humanising hospital design.

It draws on the work of the Oxford Health Arts Partnership (OHAP), an award-winning programme that delivers creative health using art and nature, for Oxford Health NHS Foundation Trust (OHFT).

Hospital patients living with dementia

Whilst many adults can cope with temporary hospitalisation for the sake of their health, older people, especially those living with dementia, can have poorer inpatient experiences and outcomes than other patient groups (Fogg *et al.* 2017). Most will be cared for in general, medical, surgical and other specialty wards: unfamiliar, hectic and noisy environments, to which individuals with cognitive impairments are much less able to adapt. Patients can become disorientated, anxious and distressed in this unfamiliar environment and function below their capability, especially when trying to communicate with nursing staff (Digby, Lee and Williams 2016). We argue, in the light of this, that not only is the quality of care provided by staff who have had continuous training in person-centred care much higher, but also that creative health interventions can enhance care. For example, staff reported in an OHAP service evaluation the observable value of creativity having a 'positive impact on patients' (Tatum, Ferrey, and Conlan 2023 p.11). Additionally, OHAP is currently developing induction training including person-centred care for all Creative Practitioners before they enter the ward and other environments.

The benefits of arts in hospitals

There is a growing research literature about the contribution of creative health to improving the health and wellbeing of patients living with dementia in acute hospitals (Boyce *et al.* 2018). Evidence is strongest for music, which benefits patients, visitors and staff (Daykin *et al.* 2018) and reduces rates of patient agitation (Pedersen *et al.* 2017). Live music is the most prevalent form of participatory arts in hospitals (Digby *et al.* 2018).

Musicians often engage with patients at their bedsides, playing requests that spark memories and initiate conversation and connecting with the individual behind the illness, which is particularly beneficial for older adults (van der Wal-Huisman 2023). They may also perform in small groups in a central open space or dayroom. Hospital arts programmes organise regular concerts and participatory music sessions that enable older patients, visitors and staff to socialise in the hospital or in its gardens. Individualised playlists can also help reduce agitation (Hanna, Chan and Maddison 2023). Playlist for Life (BBC 2019) can help families and friends co-produce these with patients.

Dance (to music) is offered for many older patients in hospitals. As a well-tolerated approach to exercise, benefits include improved communication, creativity and self-expression, balance and coordination, strength, breathing and falls reduction, and reduced agitation and anxiety (Bungay *et al.* 2022, Sport Industry Research Centre 2020). Community dance artists work with individuals and groups who are ambulant and create opportunities for chair- or bed-based work; scarves and other props are often used to enhance the positive effects of sensory and social stimulation. As with all creative arts, it is important that the art form is individually meaningful and culturally appropriate.

Dr Roosa Leimu-Brown, dancer-in-residence with OHAP, enabled patients to share positive memories and their feelings with her. During a dance session at the bedside of one patient, she noted that a grateful patient said to her, '"You are a gift." That definitely made my day! It was also lovely how each song led into a chat about a specific memory that then led into the next song' (Murray 2022 p.4). Figure 10.1 is a still from a film about OHAP's work, which can be seen at www.oxfordhealth.charity/news/art-making-a-difference.

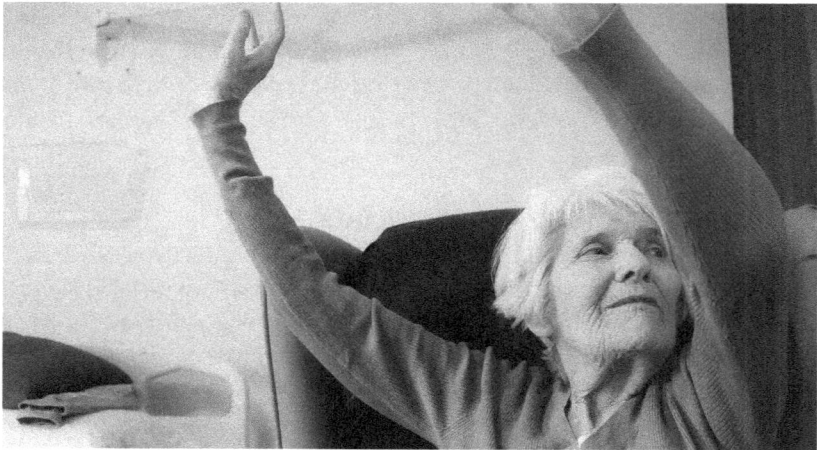

Figure 10.1 A patient dancing with Dr Roosa Leimu-Brown
CREDIT: EMMA SPELLMAN

Hospital arts programmes

In the UK, there are some 200 hospital arts programmes. Many are funded by hospital charities, and some directly by hospital trusts. Whilst individual hospital programmes vary in emphasis, all provide a wide range of creative arts programmes that aim to support the health and wellbeing needs of patients, staff and visitors. Some large NHS hospital trusts in UK cities host hospital arts teams of two or three staff, but many are run by a single part-time arts manager.

Many arts managers are members of the National Arts in Hospital Network (NAHN), a network of hospital arts managers that was relaunched under NHS Charities Together in 2024 to provide much-needed support and networking opportunities to members. NAHN's first publications, funded by Arts Council England, will be a set of comprehensive online resources to provide guidelines and support on best practice for arts in hospitals.

The work of the hospital arts manager is unique but will generally include:

- commissioning participatory arts projects for patients on wards and in waiting areas
- developing creative projects for staff to support their wellbeing
- commissioning artists to create artwork for public spaces in hospitals, waiting areas, gardens, wards and staff rooms, often integrating artwork into new build or refurbishment programmes, and appointing artists to advise on colour, finishes and furniture, usually accompanied by an engagement programme with staff and patients to ensure the artwork meets their needs
- curating temporary exhibitions of artwork
- commissioning arts resources for patients and staff.

Some arts managers also incorporate their own artistic genres through co-production and collaboration.

Good practice in hospital arts

Arts managers are also part of the creative process, and many have a background in the arts. They can support Creative Practitioners to navigate healthcare administrative systems, introducing them to different staff roles and responsibilities, risk, team dynamics and medical and nursing terminology.

Patient safety is paramount hence Creative Practitioners must be properly contracted through the NHS hospital trust Non-Medical Honorary Contract process, which can be lengthy. Creative Practitioners will need to have Safeguarding Training and be cleared through the Disclosure and Barring Service to ensure they are safe to work with vulnerable adults and children. They will need to learn to assess, mitigate and manage risks associated with using creative arts to work with frail and vulnerable individuals with complex needs. The ability to manage ever-changing risk is an essential skill. Health and safety training will also include infection control; when planning sessions, practitioners must take account of the need to wipe objects clean and ensure printed matter is single-use or encapsulated. Most teams have artist toolkits and online training to support artists.

Stepping onto a ward for the first time...

Creative Practitioners require many of the core skills and knowledge set out in Chapter 2 but in a unique combination given the need to ensure their work is person-centred, safe and attuned to health and ward cultures and hospital regulations regarding art on the ward. They need to work as part of a team that will have expectations of their professional conduct in much the same way as for a Creative Arts Therapist (CAT) or Allied Health Professional (AHP). Creative Practitioners are more likely to be supported by Health Care Assistants (HCAs), nursing cadets and approved mental health professionals. Creative therapy support posts are also being created in some NHS trusts.

On the ward, Creative Practitioners need to be able to:

- adapt to very busy and noisy environments and to fluctuations in patient cognitive health, mental state and mood by improvising their session plans, sometimes rapidly
- make empathic warm relationships with patients, beginning with active listening techniques to understand their needs
- communicate verbally and non-verbally while creating a safe space for patients to express themselves
- negotiate with other staff competing for patient time
- understand and work with the patient's perspective. They may not have considered engaging with the arts before or not participated in an art form since school. Whilst some may participate in creative arts to address boredom, others may lack confidence or willingness to engage:

> An artist may have begun with an agenda of how to bring their art form into the hospital setting, but they were then acting very much adaptably with however patients or the ward presented on any given day. This reflects the ability of the artists to adapt and develop in their role but also on the real need patients have for that quality of attention in a hospital setting, particularly where hospital staff are so stretched in coping with the physical requirements of hospital life. This quality of attention and engagement from the artist as we have said lifted spirits and any improvement in reducing stress and feeling connected to others can really benefit physiological health and patient outcomes. (Murray 2022 p.5)

Given the challenges of working in hospitals, this work is best delivered by Creative Practitioners who have experience of arts in healthcare settings and can demonstrate work of a high quality. The skills and knowledge required for this work are different from those of a professional experienced in their art form, as working with vulnerable older adults often calls for softer skills that are harder to teach: kindness, empathy, patience, positivity, sensitivity and flexibility.

Figure 10.2 is a still from a film about OHAP's work, which can be seen at www.oxfordhealth.charity/news/art-making-a-difference.

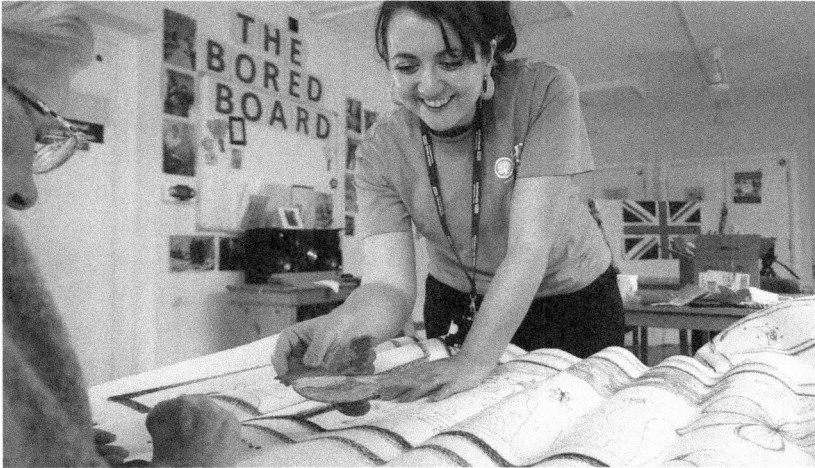

Figure 10.2 *A patient participating in an art session with artist Dionne Freeman*
CREDIT: EMMA SPELLMAN

Arts for staff wellbeing

Hospital ward staff play a key role in liaising with Creative Practitioners about patient health and changes that might affect interaction and participation, as well as identifying new admissions and/or discharges. Although the work pressures associated with prioritisation of instrumental tasks, physical care and administrative routines are challenging, at OHAP we have established good working relationships with staff and now have good staff participation in creative sessions. It can take time to create culture change but the benefits to the patient once this is established are measurable. Practitioners can also release clinical staff time and have oversight of patients while in the activity, with other hospital staff. They may also help ensure patients wear glasses, have a working hearing aid in place, are seated comfortably in a chair or get to a venue using a frame or wheelchair.

Healthcare professionals may not always be in the room with the Creative Practitioners, but they can hear and see sessions taking place and notice the impact on patients' health and wellbeing, often reporting on the positive perceptions of the value of arts interventions (Wilson 2016). The value of stimulation and the lifting of patient mood cannot be underestimated. For example, an evaluation of the OHAP arts programme in Oxfordshire Community Hospitals found not only anecdotal evidence from staff of an increase in positive mood from patients following participation in music, dance and painting sessions but also '[t]he richest data source collected throughout the interventions was the ArtsObs scores' (Tatum *et al.* 2023 p.7). Use of the Arts Observational Scale (Fancourt and Poon 2016) measured the specific impact of the intervention on patients themselves (pre and post). Significantly, 72% of participants had calm or negative moods pre-intervention, while 94% (N = 51) reported a positive mood following the intervention (Tatum *et al.* 2023).

In a separate study, an Oxfordshire Health NHS Foundation Trust (OHFT) senior matron called the arts programme: 'Therapeutic Joy' having noted the 'sheer joy patients get from it', remarking 'very significant changes' through the 'joy of possibility'; by the end the difference is clearly visible, 'they are different people by the end of the session, their mood changes from closed to open, and that makes our life on the wards much easier and more pleasurable' (Oxfordshire Health Arts Partnership 2021).

The impact of music often lifts moods for several hours after the activity, and staff report that patients are calmer and eat better. Music can also reach patients who may be otherwise unresponsive. Staff often report seeing a patient who may seem otherwise uncommunicative making small movements: tapping a finger or moving their head to the beat of the music. Musicians see this too:

> A couple of nurses...saw me sing 'Somewhere over the rainbow' to an elderly gentleman who seemed to have difficulty in speaking and communicating at first. His face lit up when he heard the music and he clapped and waved at me at the end of the song. The nurses told me that it was the most interaction they had seen from him since he had been in hospital. (Ward musician)

The therapeutic joy of the arts extends to staff, who often dance, clap or sing to the music. Joy is infectious, and staff transmit their mood to patients, and vice versa. Creative Practitioners working on wards can do much to support staff in helping foster engagement with the work, even though this is not their primary function. It helps patients living with dementia, and others, experience activities that are fundamentally non-medical; staff can see patients and relate to them in different ways that give them something to talk about with them afterwards. This was certainly the case during the COVID-19 pandemic, when many activities went online (where staff support was vital) or were channelled by arts packs and through arts activity booklets.

Arts and humanising hospital design

Most people who have been hospital patients will relate to the notion of an acute hospital as a 'city within a city' (Bates 2018). An institution that, whilst not a *total* institution (Goffman 1968), provides building-based services for diagnosis, treatment and care in ways that can be viewed as institutional. Thus, people admitted *become* patients, whose daily lives are formally managed by healthcare practices and technologies that largely limit their individuality, autonomy and agency whilst they remain on characterless, functional wards (relatively) isolated from society.

The negative impact of hospital design and totalising practice has long been recognised, and proposals to counterbalance 'inhuman' aspects include not only improving the built environment but also facilitating visual stimulation and access to nature, arts and gardens (Bates 2018). Part of The King's Fund Enhancing the Healing Environment (EHE) programme 2000–2006 to address the adverse effects of hospital buildings on patient, staff and visitor health focused on supportive design for people with dementia. Recommendations included the use of spatial design to improve self-confidence and promote activity and night-time sleep, as well as artwork to humanise the institutional feel of a hospital ward and aid navigation in an unfamiliar building (Waller, Masterson and Finn 2013).

Besides being aesthetically pleasing, artwork in hospitals is art with a purpose. It fosters social interaction, aids memory, lifts mood and complements and supports patient treatment goals, whilst supporting staff. Art makes hospitals calm and positive spaces for families and friends.

Conclusion

Creative health practice is in the vanguard of ongoing work to 'humanise' hospitals (Bates 2018), enabling people living with dementia to have an improved hospital experience with better outcomes. This chapter offers guidance to Creative Practitioners about how their work can help to meet the physiological, emotional, psychosocial and cultural needs for patients living with the condition in these environments. It is not without significant challenges; however, the rewards of hospital-based arts practice are very considerable, and this chapter is a contribution to improving it further.

LEARNING POINTS

- Training and development: Learn about values-based person-centred care practices, and access and complete a dementia awareness course – ask your arts manager to signpost resources.

- Cultivate good relationships with all ward staff including ancillary workers, as they provide information about how patients are feeling, new patients and visitors who also need support.

- Find a peer mentor, an experienced arts practitioner who is working in or has worked in hospital settings, via the arts manager who commissioned you.

- Keep a reflective journal and take time to record and reflect on your relationships with patients and staff and the impact on the unique culture of a busy NHS hospital and ward.

- Harness your soft skills to express kindness, empathy, patience, positivity, sensitivity and flexibility in your person-centred practices.

References

Bates, V. (2018) '"Humanising" healthcare environments: Architecture, arts and design in modern hospitals.' *Design for Health* 2, 1, 5–19.

BBC (British Broadcasting Corporation) (2019) Playlist for life. www.playlistforlife.org.uk/resources

Boyce, M., Bungay, H., Munn-Giddings, C. and Wilson, C. (2018) 'The impact of the arts in healthcare on patients and service users: A critical review.' *Health and Social Care in the Community* 26, 4, 458–473.

Bungay, H., Hughes, S., Jacobs, C. and Zhang, J. (2022) 'Dance for health: The impact of creative dance sessions on older people in an acute hospital setting.' *Arts & Health* 14, 1, 1–13.

Daykin, N., Parry, B., Ball, K., Walters, D. *et al.* (2018) 'The role of participatory music making in supporting people with dementia in hospital environments.' *Dementia* 17, 6, 686–701.

Digby, R., Lee, S. and Williams, A. (2016) 'The experience of people with dementia and nurses in hospital: An integrative review.' *Journal of Clinical Nursing* 26, 9–10, 1152–1171.

Fancourt, D. and Poon, M. (2016) 'Validation of the Arts Observational Scale (ArtsObS) for the evaluation of performing arts activities in health care settings.' *Arts & Health: An International Journal for Research, Policy and Practice* 8, 2, 140–153.

Fogg, C., Meredith, P., Bridges, J., Gould, G. P. and Griffiths, P. (2017) 'The relationship between cognitive impairment, mortality and discharge characteristics in a large cohort of older adults with unscheduled admissions to an acute hospital: A retrospective observational study.' *Age and Ageing* 46, 5, 794–780.

Goffman, E. (1968) *Asylums: Essays on the Social Situation of Mental Patients and Other Inmates.* Harmondsworth: Penguin.

Hanna, S., Chan, L. and Maddison, J. (2023) 'Can a personalised music listening intervention decrease agitation in hospitalised patients with dementia? A feasibility trial.' *Frontiers in Psychiatry* 14, 1186043.

Murray, C. (2022) *Impact Report for Regular Arts Provision at Witney Community Hospital.* www.oxfordhealth.charity/Handlers/Download.ashx?IDMF=36f1209c-d88a-4f33-bcc1-c4290fd67258

Oxfordshire Health Arts Partnership (2021) Evaluation report: making a difference through our artists-in-residence. Oxford Health NHS Foundation Trust and Oxford Health Charity. www.oxfordhealth.charity/news/making-a-difference-artists?tirle=making-a-difference-artists

Pedersen, S., Andersen, P., Lugo, R., Andreassen, M. and Sütterlin, S. (2017) 'Effects of music on agitation in dementia: A meta-analysis.' *Frontiers in Psychology* 8, 742.

Sport Industry Research Centre (2020) *Dance to Health 'Phase 1 Roll-Out [Test And Learn]' Evaluation: Final Report.* Sheffield: Sheffield Hallam University, Sport Industry Research Centre. https://ae-sop.org/wp-content/uploads/sites/63/2020/06/DANCE-TO-HEALTH-evaluation-by-SHU-SIRC-final-report-May-2020.pdf

Tatum, M., Ferrey, D. and Conlan, A. (2023) *Arts Impact Measured: A Service Evaluation of OHAP Arts-in-Health Interventions.* Oxford Health Charity. www.oxfordhealth.charity/Handlers/Download.ashx?IDMF=73ddccfd-c355-413b-9553-e25738de8235

Van der Wal-Huisman, H., van den Berg, N. M., Paans, W., Bezold, L. *et al.* (2023) 'Live bedside music for hospitalized older adults: A qualitative descriptive interview study.' *International Journal of Older People Nursing 18,* e12574.

Waller, S., Masterson, A. and Finn, H. (2013) *Developing Supportive Design for People with Dementia. The King's Fund's Enhancing the Healing Environment Programme 2009–2012.* London: Kings Fund. https://assets.kingsfund.org.uk/f/256914/x/7895f8facd/developing_supportive_design_people_with_dementia_2013.pdf

Wilson, C. (2016) 'Healthcare professionals' perceptions of the value and impact of the arts in healthcare settings: A critical review of the literature.' *International Journal of Nursing Studies 56,* 90–101.

CHAPTER 11

Moving Kinship *with* Dementia

A Feminist More-than-Human Practice

Beatrice Allegranti

As I walk through the corridors of the care home, I hear familiar singing from a distant communal room – '*Que Sera Sera*'. I'm caught in a temporal flux, a present-past (Allegranti 2024, Braidotti 2022). Everyone here is my parent's generation, and I think of them now, how they used to sing me this generational song and that they are no longer alive; perhaps I'm searching. Here, in the intimacy of people's rooms, I meet residents and engage in poetic conversations. As both choreographer and psychotherapist, I listen with attention to the *movements* of lives. People talk with an unquestioning openness, and I glimpse into lives endured during apartheid South Africa: *Mandela was a wonderful man. Incredible inspiration*. Or those who toiled in Yorkshire coal mines: *You had to be strong, strong as a family too*. A woman, who chose childlessness, stands as the sole survivor of her lineage: *I'm the last one. Where am I going to go?* While a grandmother basks in the abundance of generations that visit and holds them dear: *It's a good feeling to hold them there. I love you to the moon and back*. I meet a woman moving with stealth along the corridor, her walking frame becoming prosthetic legs, and I learn that her kinship is with an exquisite murmuration of starlings. Together our wingspan opens in a fleeting, yet coordinated improvisational dance:

> *I'm still there*
> *The last Starling*
> *Yeah, yeah, yeah, yeah*
> *Fly like a bird*
> *This is my real life*
> *Wonderful life*

Love flying
Friends can be like family.

In another room, as a woman brushes her hair, I hear about collective kinship, communities bound by mutual support, where kin is extended beyond family ties serving as an unwavering anchor:

If they hadn't got it, somebody else had it
We were a community
Community
It was lovely to have that privilege, to grow in that sense
Because if you haven't got it, they have it
Community, not only your family, but wider community.

Community, from the Latin genesis *with unity*. This is a home, a care home where each person is paradoxically together-alone. I listen to voices of resistance, of collectivity, of reckoning, of abundance, isolation, grief and mourning. How can we move *with* unity in dementia care? One of the care staff leads me to a door. Through it, I see an elderly man slumped in an armchair, immobile, perhaps asleep; he has no visitors. This member of the care team tells me, 'He's a homosexual and doesn't have any family.' I linger in the doorway, my breathing becomes unsteady, my own body sinks and concaves with the feeling about this microcosm of societal bias; the walls of this care home are porous. Equally, the medicalisation of dementia framed as a pathological condition, while intended to reduce stigma and taboo, has often resulted in more stigmatisation. A biomedical bias emphasises cognitive deterioration where dementia is depicted as a devastating 'loss of self' or even loss of humanity. A hypercognitive model of dementia equates the notion of 'self' with mental function and language residing within bodies as 'containers' (Post 2000) and does not take into account personal and social experiences, where it is understood that affect – the embodied feeling and force of a relational event – endures (Allegranti 2019 2024, Stern 2010 p.8). Within this complex milieu, the lives of partners, children, parents, friends and carers are impacted, and a newly embodied way of relating must be found for all; if not, the impact of a dementia diagnosis and way of life will be a traumatising legacy.

Homeward bound, driving along the motorway, my hands tightly grip the steering wheel. I loosen, take a breath, regulate my nervous system and think about what we hold onto in this life, what we allow ourselves to move *with* and the traces that we leave behind. The refrains of people living with dementia and their carers find their way into this writing: anxieties, hopes, fears, dreams cherished or unrealised; people and places mourned, they all form an indelible connection to a future-present (Barad 2007, Braidotti 2022), a transgenerational opportunity to time-travel with dementia and inherit the future and past all at once. This writing is a practice of *moving* kinship across the page and of putting feminisms to work by situating personal human experiences of dementia within wider, complex, more-than-human social, geo-political and environmental processes, in which we are inextricably entangled. To ignore these tangles risks dehumanising people living with dementia and reproducing (at worst) oppressive systemic structures of relating.

Moving Kinship

Moving Kinship©, a feminist transdisciplinary practice, unfolds in diverse UK and global hubs such as arts centres, theatres, museums, libraries, hospitals, private homes, care homes and grassroots organisations, often giving rise to full-scale artistic works (see Allegranti 2024). Collaborating with an international artistic team, I engage intergenerationally with families affected by early onset dementia, older adults living with dementia, youth environmental activists, LGBTQ+ communities and activists and Black feminist activists, as well as artists and scientists across the world. Each hub creatively moves kinship in trauma-responsive ways with each community, striving to expand a window of tolerance – the regulatory capacity to recognise and stay present with unsettling affect. By working *with* the 'trouble' of individual, family, community or kinship groups, the hubs offer an opening for applying feminist ethics, for engaging with and navigating traumatic loss and dispossession, grief, mourning and the embodied and embedded politics of the unseen and unheard.

The established transdisciplinary methodology includes creating bespoke live and digital performances *with* and *for* diverse audiences, fostering collaboration, collectivity and micro-cultures of belonging and care (*ibid.* pp.29–56). These performances act as 'matrixial kin' (*ibid.* pp.47–48), capturing the affective nuance of kinship through conversation, transgenerational stories, gestures, micro-movements and song. Kinship thus expands beyond immediate family ties to other families, communities, individuals and the artistic team, and with the performance material itself.

Dementia disrupts traditional kinship, compelling me to reckon with its tenuous and shifting movements. *Listening with movement* (Allegranti 2024 p.33) is a central methodological refrain and is part of my *kin*-aesthetic attention. *Kin*-aesthesia is the new word I have created to include:

> ...three imbricated aspects: the sense of movement (including proprioceptive and interoceptive or sensory motor aspects), the vital role of aesthetics in

forming movement (in both choreographic and psychotherapy practices), and the emergent material kinship – and ethics and politics therein – during the process of human and more-than human movement relating. (Allegranti 2024 p.10)

Allowing for the simultaneity of these layers as a process of *listening with movement* challenges the limits of 20th-century anthropocentric humanism, which is predicated on separation and binaries such as body/mind, nature/culture and subjective/objective, and maintains the long-held view of the bodies as solely human and as discrete (individual) entities. Instead, my feminist new materialist discussion emphasises the 'more-than-human': a de-centring of the human as the driver for transformation and resituating a relational view of bodies as ongoing *kin*-aesthetic processes, never neutral, that are in Karen Barad's terms 'entangled' within the complexities of culture, politics, history, technology and the environment (Allegranti 2019, 2024, Barad 2007, Braidotti 2022).

As a white intersectional feminist, influenced by the germinal work of Audre Lorde (2017, 1988/2017, 1984/2007) and Kimberlé Crenshaw (1989, 1991), I extend awareness of and accountability for body politics in my practice: not only for sexualities and genders but also for race, class, age and disability. I recognise my own embodied intersections of privilege and oppression and cannot escape my internalised racism, ableism, misogyny and homophobia (Allegranti 2024). Cultivating a *kin*-aesthetic practice maintains accountability and is foundational for inclusive and equitable relating.

The writing below diffracts (Allegranti 2024, Barad 2007, Haraway 2016) multiple experiences and voices: a care home resident living with dementia, their spouse, four professional dancers and the emergent choreographic and bespoke performance material with its more-than-human evocations. These interwoven insights offer critically conscious and feminist *kin*-aesthetic learning points for dementia care.

Baobab

The three of us are seated in armchairs facing each other, in a care home communal area. Chris and Jane are a white South African couple in their late 60s. Chris lives with dementia, and as soon as I introduce myself, he clearly states his preference and perhaps his limits: *I want to listen*. I want to listen-with Chris, and in doing so, to excavate the micro-movements of kinship behind, underneath and alongside our relating. Chris's meaningful statement of listening makes itself felt in his shifting micro-movements. The chair is becoming a place of discomfort for him, it seems to be ill-fitting for his long limbs; he is restless, unseated. To unseat is a verb, a movement removing him from power. I notice my own bodily response: irregular breathing and increased heart rate, I'm becoming uneasy in my listening, agitated. My body forms into dysregulation: a hypo-aroused (dorsal ventral) freeze of my sympathetic nervous system (Porges 2011, Rothschild 2017); and I become curious about what/who is 'freezing' or dissociating. I reorganise myself internally, shift position and take an audible out breath so that I can keep listening. As the conversation continues, Jane's words reveal a tangled affect: *It's hard to hold it all together*, and then I land, my body grounded as the weight of dementia enters the relationship.

Trauma-responsive work is about noticing what lands in your body and how it lands in intersectional bodies in different and more-than-human ways. I learn that Chris and Jane grew up in post-war Apartheid South Africa, and I am wary about how the biases will unravel, where the ruptures will make themselves felt. Then I hear about Jane's expansive kinship:

> *I was born in Malawi*
> *I was the first white child born in a chief's territory*
> *and was adopted into his tribe*
> *They'd come on my birthday every year*
> *Wouldn't it be extraordinary if they were to just walk in now?*
> *They've remembered me.*

Extended losses reverberate in this room, fracturing kinship as dementia weaves with cultural bodies. Life now, marked by unbearable ordinariness, finds Jane working as a supermarket cashier, whilst Chris lives in this care home. Being-with this layered legacy foregrounds an ethics of relating, echoing Sara Ahmed and Judith Butler's considerations not only on what constitutes a grievable life but also what is (socio-politically) considered a liveable life in the first place (Butler 2010, Ahmed 2014). Inter-human hierarchies persist, marginalising dis-abled bodies, Black bodies, LGBTQ+ bodies, women's bodies to varying degrees of liveability and grievability. How do intersecting oppressions and privileges shape the perceived liveability and grievability for those living with dementia and their family carers? In our unspoken yet palpably affecting conversation, the traumatic oppression of racism intertwines with white privilege and intersects with dementia.

Chris's restlessness resurfaces and he interjects: *No! Not like that.* Jane mentions his regular 'outbursts', uttered as if he's not present. I turn to face Chris directly, ensuring his presence is acknowledged, sensing his frustration at being unable to freely participate in the telling of his own story, the disempowering sense of being unable to grasp his memories. With an affirming tone, I prompt,

Tell me more about the Baobab. The tree, fleetingly mentioned earlier, now evokes its more-than-human presence within this innocuous communal 'living' room:

> *It grows very slowly*
> *Full of water*
> *Animals like elephants if they're desperate will try to get water*
> *It's colossal.*

I experience another landing in my bodily response, a calmer activation of my parasympathetic (ventral vagal) nervous system (Porges 2011, Rothschild 2017). Chris also relaxes into his chair as if resting against the Baobab's expansive trunk. I recognise Jane and Chris's embodied intersectional experiences as they actively re-member – a process Donna Haraway likens to 'reprise, revive, retake, recuperate' (Haraway 2016 p.34). Re-membering is collective movement, akin to Baobab roots entwining with fungal filaments, passing resources to future generations (Simard 2022). My resolve strengthens to nurture a transgenerational *kin*-aesthetics of care in dementia, where somatic awareness highlights subtle movements – the shifting in chairs, audible breaths, the affective nuances of the (un)spoken – and recognising the agency of more-than-human actors in communication.

Feminist with-ness

In the following days, I take this intersecting material into our rehearsal for the bespoke performance. I invite Rudzani to work with the Baobab, and she roots herself, with bent knees, stable legs, her arms open, with palms facing each other. In its momentary pause, this is a powerful and iconic stance. As this choreography forms, Rudzani receives herself in the affective landscape of her own heritage as a Black South African:

> *There's a resource here all the time, it's a not fixed way of being*
> *It has a certain way, certain integration. It transforms*
> *The Baobab roots everything*
> *Each root represents every journey taken.*

This choreographic material weaves inextricably into a more-than-human kinship with the *Baobab Tree* that is our feminist 'with-ness' (Allegranti 2024 p.46) for re-routing and *integrating* the intolerable. With-ness emphasises the self-other tangle and the capacity to nurture a sense of collectivity amid the unpredictability of growing new possibilities for relating. However, expanding the capacity to with-ness in dementia care is an ethical imperative that germinates from the individual yet is powered by the collective.

Amandla Awethu/Power Is Ours, Power to the People

This bespoke performance swirls around us, the performers encircling the care home audience and reconnecting with Chris and Jane's conversation. In the care home garden, on a day in May that marked the end of 2021's final COVID-19 lockdown, our performance resonates with what Takeshi describes as the *Rite of Spring: bringing energy of the new-born*. We've transformed the garden into an open-air immersive performance space, with its slanting grass aspect, paved pathway, rose trestles and an audience of residents, care home staff and some family members. Luke notices: *It feels like family involvement. I feel like I'm in someone's house. In their garden.* Kinship with dementia leaks beyond the confines of the care home and tangles with the natural environment. Later, Luke comments on the more-than-human temporal affect of this performance: *I remember looking up at one point and thinking these trees are older than everyone. They're rocked, centred.*

In this UK care home, most carers are people of colour, while all the care home residents are white. In the audience, I see varied expressions: smiles, curiosity, confusion, tears and awe. My amplified voice contrasts sharply with the intimacy of 23 individual conversations the previous week and resonates with Aneta, Luke, Rudzani, Maria and Takeshi's movements. Their dancing intertwines with my spoken words in an ongoing material flow where neither words nor bodies are in oppositional hierarchy (Allegranti 2024, Barad 2007). Living with dementia can make listening and speaking feel like navigating an incomprehensible language. Yet shifting emphasis to movement-relating redirects the focus from speech acts towards discerning meaningful (*kin*-aesthetic) connections, opening new possibilities within this new realm of choreographing-with dementia communication.

Gradually, Rudzani's fingers sense like antennae, micro-ripples shifting through her torso, sprouting into one leg's seemingly accelerated growth. Becoming-with (Allegranti 2024, Barad 2007) the Baobab, Rudzani's shape-shifting transports her, the other dancers and the audience. Her hands are now behind her curved spine, like antennae tracking rhythmic backward steps. Focused curiosity defines Rudzani's purposeful movements – fingers, hands and arms circling, spiralling. With steady breath and soft pulsing, Rudzani re-forms her gesture into a freedom-fighting fist. The four dancers repeat in formation, mapping the garden's terrain. *Kin*-aesthetic resistance is shaping the care home, unifying bodies. Punching upwards, the fist embodies strength, determination, justice, while spiralling arms and torsos ensure continuity. Rudzani chants, echoed in call and response from us all: *Amandla Awethu/Power Is Ours, Power to the People*. Aligned, we move through the clapping audience, a collectively powered *kin*-aesthetic affirmation. I search for Chris and Jane and hear a male voice say: *I think I recognised myself but didn't want to.* A woman extends a hand, met by Luke, who admires her nail polish. Takeshi gestures towards a member of the care staff, inviting them to dance. Our performance leaves a somatic marker (Poppa and Bechara 2018), a neuro-physical trace that agitates me into recalibrating 'care' as a skilful navigation of kinship's micro-movements, challenging biases that linger within bodies and institutions, by re-forming in *kin*-aesthetic ways. Doing so stretches into a more-than-human imaginary, facilitating small acts of (relational) activism.

Dementia is more-than

Akin to the Baobab rooted for millennia, absorbing, retaining and reshaping transgenerational (more-than-human) experiences, feminist (decolonising) care seeks to ethically re-route individual and institutional bodies. Doing so response-ably (Allegranti 2024, Haraway 2016) interrupts cycles of dispossession – of not belonging to oneself or to community – through collective knowing and doing. *Moving Kinship* is a radical care practice, allowing for micro-moments of recuperation and resistance through *kin*-aesthetic means: acknowledging vulnerabilities and complicities, noticing how they land in bodies; how gestures shape and re-form. This is a practice that revives traumatic and traumatising gestures as a resource for bodying otherwise – a futuring of intimacy and contradictions, while decentring whiteness and the human as the sole drivers for transformation.

The *Moving Kinship* bespoke performance engages people living with dementia, families and caregivers inclusively and equitably, as acts of micro-activism. For me, this feminist practice entails a *kin*-aesthetic vigilance: sensitivity to the diverse intersectionality of (more-than-human) bodies and supporting a nuanced and non-oppressive sense of bodily plurality as a mode of survival, growth and re-generation in relating. This foundation creates restitution in our places of care.

Dementia is always more-than, a call to action from voices often silenced, demanding recognition of the more-than-human. As ecologically distributed, dementia teaches us to re-route in ways that are not predicated on othering. Working from this recognition is a speculative gesture for (feminist) justice, a care-full growth and recalibration, for moving-with the seemingly ineffable of dementia in more-than tolerable ways.

LEARNING POINTS

- **Listening with movement**: *Moving Kinship*© demonstrates the importance of *listening with movement* when understanding individuals living with dementia. Bespoke performance hubs encourage deeper, creative understandings of individuals living with dementia by attuning to subtle movements, sensory shifts, affective nuances and transgenerational experiences, fostering relational connection and expression for individuals, caregivers and practitioners.

- **Intersectional understanding of kinship**: Recognising the intersecting identities, including race, genders, sexualities, class and dis-ability, is crucial in understanding how dementia impacts their lived experiences. By acknowledging these intersections, caregivers and practitioners can provide more inclusive and equitable support and invite bodily plurality.

- **Feminist trauma-responsive care**: This involves acknowledging how trauma lands in different intersectional bodies in different ways, and it is an ethical priority for practitioners to learn how to navigate the relational complexities of intersecting oppressions and privileges in creative and embodied ways.

- **More-than-human understanding of dementia**: Dementia is not solely a cognitive or medical condition but a complex interplay of personal, social, political, environmental and cultural factors. Embracing a more-than-human perspective acknowledges the interconnectedness of all beings and environments involved in the care experience. This approach encourages caregivers and practitioners to consider the relational dynamics between humans, nonhuman entities and the broader ecosystem in dementia care practices.

References

Ahmed, S. (2014) *The Cultural Politics of Emotion.* Edinburgh: Edinburgh University Press.

Allegranti, B. (2019) 'Moving Kinship: Between Choreography, Performance and the More-than-Human.' In S. Prickett and H. Thomas (2019) (eds) *The Routledge Dance Handbook.* London: Routledge.

Allegranti, B. (2024) *Moving Kinship: Practicing Feminist Justice in a More-than-Human World.* Oxford/New York: Routledge.

Barad, K. (2007) *Meeting the Universe Halfway: Quantum Physics and the Entanglement of Matter and Meaning.* Durham/London: Duke University Press.

Braidotti, R. (2022) *Posthuman Feminism.* Cambridge: Polity Press.

Butler, J. (2010) *Frames of War: When Is Life Grievable?* London/New York: Verso.

Crenshaw, K. (1989) 'Demarginalizing the intersection of race and sex: A Black feminist critique of antidiscrimination doctrine, feminist theory and antiracist politics.' *University of Chicago Legal Forum 139,* 139–168.

Crenshaw, K. (1991) 'Mapping the margins: Intersectionality, identity politics, and violence against women of color.' *Stanford Law Review 43,* 6, 1241–1299.

Haraway, D. J. (2016) *Staying with the Trouble.* Durham/London: Duke University Press.

Lorde, A. (1984/2007) *Sister Outsider Essays and Speeches.* Berkeley, CA: Crossing Press.

Lorde, A. (1988/2017) *A Burst of Light and Other Essays*. New York: Ixia Press.

Lorde, A. (2017) *Your Silence Will Not Protect You: Essays and Poems*. London: Silver.

Poppa, T. and Bechara, A. (2018) 'The somatic marker hypothesis: Revisiting the role of the "body-loop" in decision-making.' *Current Opinion in Behavioral Sciences* 1, 19, 61–66.

Porges, S. (2011) *The Polyvagal Theory: Neurophysiological Foundations of Emotions, Attachment, Communication, and Self-Regulation*. New York: W.W. Norton & Company.

Post, S. G. (2000) 'The Concept of Alzheimer's Disease in a Hypercognitive Society.' In P. J. Whitehouse, K. Maurer and J. F. Ballenger (2000) (ed.) *Concepts of Alzheimer Disease*. Baltimore, MD: John Hopkins University Press.

Rothschild, B. (2017) *The Body Remembers: Revolutionising Trauma Treatment. Volume 2*. New York: W.W. Norton & Company.

Simard, S. (2022) *Finding the Mother Tree: Uncovering the Wisdom and Intelligence of the Forest*. London: Penguin.

Stern, D. N. (2010) *Forms of Vitality: Exploring Dynamic Experience in Psychology and the Arts*. Oxford: Oxford University Press.

CHAPTER 12

Still Climbing Mountains

A Conversation on Creativity, Aspiration and Living with Dementia

Ronald Amanze and David Truswell

Ronald Amanze is a record producer living with dementia. David Truswell is an independent writer and researcher on dementia and its impact on Black, Asian and minority ethnic communities. Over a number of years, Ronald and David have collaborated on a variety of projects to raise awareness about dementia and involve people living with dementia in creative projects and have now set up Dementia in Dub, a community interest company that develops and runs intergenerational creative arts and music projects with people living with dementia.

In this chapter, Ronald talks to David about the importance of creativity and the crucial part it has played in him managing his life after a stroke and the onset of dementia. Ronald found his voice through writing 'The Mountains I Still Climb' and joining a self-directed group who write and post online Dementia Diaries, which empowered him to use his music-producing skills to co-produce and co-facilitate creative dementia awareness through the Photobook and the Box of Smiles projects, all of which inspired the book he wrote with David. In 'The Mountains I Still Climb', Ronald reflects on his experience of living with dementia and how, through poetry and music, he became an artist and dementia activist with a renewed sense of agency and purpose in the world.

DT How is creativity important for you, Ronald?

RA You mean why is my music activity and my poetry activity important? I find it essential. I've always been around the music world, and I've always loved music. But I didn't realise that music was what I needed as a form of medication. I didn't realise that writing my thoughts and feelings down could be described as poetry and art. I didn't realise how important these would be in rescuing me at a time when I was so anxious, so depressed, so frustrated with conversations about something that mattered to me but not being listened to and not being heard. I didn't realise how much of an outlet music, poetry and art were as well as making me feel heard.

DT Can you say a bit about how you became a Dementia Diarist?

RA Dementia Diaries is part of the creative thing that rescued me. The first Dementia Diary I wrote was 'The Mountains I Still Climb'. I wrote at a time when I was just finding everything about the care and support system, and all these people I suddenly found in my life, frustrating. It was astonishing that for all the conversations I was having with them and all their good intentions to try and support me, nothing ever came out of it. I just found them trying to make me a vehicle or item on their agenda.

Once, I wanted to do a charity record for a dementia charity. I said this is how I'd like to go about it, and this is the plan. When they came back to me, they had reduced my plan to something almost invisible. Suddenly my idea became their idea, and they incorporated it into their local programme. That totally destroyed me because I put so much enthusiasm, excitement and vision into something they totally trivialised and then deleted me from the whole picture that I painted. So, I wrote a letter to the head of that organisation and said, 'You come to see me, but you don't see *me*.'

DT So that experience was what you turned into that first Dementia Diary entry, 'The Mountains I Still Climb'?

RA Absolutely. I suppose there were other influences that led to me writing 'The Mountains I Still Climb' but that was the specific circumstance which was just full of frustration and exhaustion. I find it amazing how something I wrote at one of my lowest moments suddenly became referred to as art.

DT So how did you connect up with Dementia Diaries from there?

RA Well David, you invited me to an event in Brighton where initially I couldn't get in because it was very late to get any funding, but I decided to go down anyway.

While I was there, I made myself busy by looking at the stalls like everybody else and I met somebody from Dementia Diaries. When I went to their stand, they said, 'Do you want to get involved?' When I looked at it, I said, 'This ain't for me is it? It's more for different communities because there's no one like me here, is there?' Then this guy said to me, 'Well if you don't get involved how can we ever have anybody like you in the mix of things?'

We spoke for a little while and because he was so joyful and pleasant to speak to, I came back and followed up the connection by sending 'The Mountains I Still Climb', saying, 'Here you are. Use this as a Dementia Diary.' And that's what they did.

DT You went from strength to strength with Dementia Diaries, didn't you?

RA It's amazing that something I wrote when I was sad and depressed is now being referred to as art. Because it wasn't art to me. It was my way of communicating and sharing my thoughts and realising that sometimes we have to camouflage our communications, especially when we speak culturally, because otherwise it would be interpreted as being aggressive or too loud. When you do it in a creative way it becomes more than what is defined by assumptions. It becomes art.

Through art you can express everything about your existence. You can be open, you can cry, shed all your tears and anxieties and not be crucified for it. Also, when it comes out of you, it leaves you with a bad, sad feeling that you have done something wrong. But when I write my feelings down on paper and mix it in a song for instance, I can come back to that feeling. I can reflect on what I've written, then I cherish it. It becomes art. I look at it and think, 'Whoa, I'm glad I wrote that.' I can marvel over it.

I often marvel over 'The Mountains I Still Climb' because it is a beautiful piece of work. You encouraged me to appreciate it and recognise the beauty in it. You kept on about it and I now love it as a piece of art, not as an expression of sadness and frustration. So, art can regenerate your emotions and your feelings. Give me medication and that puts me to sleep but give me art and I start to sing, I start to dance. Even if I'm talking about something that is too much for me to handle, I can still do it with a song. I get a lot of satisfaction from reflecting on things I have written that at the time were just too much for me to bear, and now it's what brings so much joy to my thoughts. It strengthens me as being someone who wasn't an artist before, but I am one now. I was involved with artists before, I was involved with music and all of that. But I wasn't an artist. Now I am.

I get invited to recite and perform things I have written and would have ordinarily discarded. Art dignifies you. My music and my writing for therapy has dignified me. It made me, in some quarters, someone who is considered a person who is more than just someone with a dementia diagnosis and of limited capacity. I know that what I do has given me a level of regard that I would not have had before because I'm now seen as creative. I'm now seen as an artist. Even though they may not give me that title they see me now in some respects as someone who has more brains than they thought I had. Often people say to me, 'Where did you get educated?' and I didn't get educated. If anything, I got educated in Wormwood Scrubs on my life journey. It also motivates me to want to live more, to say more and do more.

Because when you are involved in the creative process, it makes you become inquisitive and curious about things. Things I wasn't inquisitive or curious about and I now am. When I hear other people talking, the art side of me opens up to look at things differently. When people talk about their feelings and emotions, it's a vehicle that enables me to share my feelings, to live with my diagnosis without the sadness. Because I can mix it with a song, and I can also associate myself with a lot of other like-minded people. What that did was introduce me to a wider community living in harmony and also peer support.

DT I think that links up with some of the other things you have been doing to help other people be more creative such as the Photobook Project and the Box of Smiles.

RA It's so easy not to have a purpose after health issues. It's about whatever you can continue to do in life nine times out of ten regardless of what your disability is. It's that thing where you can share different moments, and you can do things and be adventurous. Even though I started with the writing, it also made me appreciative of art. Art for me encompasses everything. Like the Photobook Project, that was just a natural thing for me and now I'm an artist. I appreciate art in every respect.

DT The Photobook Project involved taking a picture of your world every day, and you were part of the pilot, not only as one of the early subjects but also as part of the development board. We sent out cameras to people from various communities to take pictures of their world every day that were turned into a book from each participant.

RA The Photobook Project, for me, was just remarkable. Absolutely. I started to appreciate things visually. I'd look out of my window and I'm looking at how to interpret and understand, what is a tree or a brick wall? How do I take a picture of that wall and put some words on it or put some creative talk to it? I'd have to tell people, 'I hit a brick wall, but guess what? The wall fell down!' It made me give different terms to lots of things.

The Photobook Project was the first one, that was the first type of thing for me. Creativity in all its different forms is what I'm all about. I need it. It rescues me. It allows me to be unruly. An unruly mind that sometimes can be overwhelmed by impulses really can cherish art. Art is good for unruly minds. The sort of mind that is leaning towards anxiety, stress or whatever. Give that person a paintbrush, or a pen, or a camera.

DT That includes everybody doesn't it? Where we have done the Box of Smiles, asking people to write a few lines about what a smile means to them, people have said, 'I can't do that...'.

RA Yes, at the time people have said, 'I can't do that', 'I'm not gonna do that', whatever. And when they do it, they become possessive about it. 'It's mine!' And I say, 'Yeah, it's yours. But didn't you say you didn't want to do it?' And actually, it's a beautiful thing. It cuts through a lot of embarrassment and discomfort once it's done. Box of Smiles is a simple conversation that can be so powerful when embraced or captured in a smile.

DT I remember the guy at the event in Teignmouth who said it was the sort of thing he would get asked to do at school and said it never works and he would never be able to do it, yet in the workshop he was up at the front of everyone reciting his poem.

RA At first, he looked like he was going to be a troublemaker, and after we had the session, he became like a friend! He was around us afterwards upstairs and talking, and that was more than we expected. And he started to talk about his life. There are so many people who say, 'I don't write poems. I don't want to do this. No, that's not for me.' That's art. It helps you discover things that were dormant within you. It helps you deal with things.

DT When we've done the Box of Smiles with a group of people, when everybody has said what makes them smile, it changes the whole atmosphere in the room.

RA Absolutely, we saw that when we did the workshop in Ladbroke Grove – there was a lady who was very determined to be of a certain (uncooperative) way and then she becomes the keenest person to be a contributor and just kept on talking about her memories. It just takes you places, joyfully. They didn't remember the beating they may have gotten growing up or the troubles they may have had, they were just remembering good things.

From what I understand it's alright to embrace your shortcomings. I worked out for myself very quickly, 'Ronald, nine times out of ten when you speak you ramble on, you lose direction and you just might need a translator.' But with art you don't really need a translator.

DT That reminds me of one of the Photobooks created by a Chinese lady who does not speak English anymore, but you could look at her Photobook and realise that you didn't need a translator because you could see what she was seeing.

RA Yes that's it perfectly. With art I don't need a translator. There's a lot of translation that needs to be done for people who have got dementia because they are tackling assumptions. I think some people living with dementia could be amazing creators. Anyone can be creative, but I've seen some work that people are doing now in terms of art, and I think, 'Wow!'

It's what I need and it's what I'm going to nurture on my journey through this dementia thing. The biggest thing that keeps me going is creative expression through art. Art makes me breathe. It helps me breathe without embarrassment. It helps me reflect on life without regret. It makes me gravitate towards beautiful conversations. It really works for me.

If it wasn't for art, I may have vanished by now. I know this as a fact. I would have disappeared. I would have become silent. I would never have been seen. I would have never been recognised as someone who had feelings and thoughts and aspirations. I would have been totally deleted from the radar by exclusion.

What has led to me being excluded, albeit briefly and occasionally? Nine times out of ten, people in my world, and my tendency to be emotionally excited, pushed me aside as being aggressive or being someone whose attitude should be medicated. Instead, what has brought me to the attention of some agencies has been the fact that I have been involved with arts-related and creative-related activities, and if I didn't have those, what would I have had? I would have had a dementia diagnosis. Art has made me visible and given me a voice where I had no voice.

THE MOUNTAINS I STILL CLIMB

You come to see me
But you don't see me
We have a conversation
But you don't hear me
And I've been thinking
If you don't hear me
How you gonna know what I'm thinking?
Your eyes fixed on me
Sometimes you smile
I always smile
And I wonder if you know why

But if you don't hear me
When I'm speaking
How you gonna know what I'm thinking?
And if you can't hear me
When I'm calling
How you gonna know
That I'm falling?
And though I no longer
Dance beneath quiet skies
Nor run across open fields
I wonder if you'd believe
The mountains I still climb?

(AMANZE 2019)

LEARNING POINTS

All practitioners, including creative arts practitioners working with people living with dementia, should be asking themselves the following questions:

- What aspects of my (your) practice enable people to maintain creativity in their lives?

- How does my (your) practice respect and include opportunities for people to exercise existing professional skills if they wish to?

- How does my (your) practice seek to understand and respond to people's cultural needs and creative aspirations?

Resources

Amanze, R. (2019) 'The Mountains I Still Climb.' Dementia Diaries with Ronald Amanze. https://dementiadiaries.org/entry/10124/the-mountains-i-still-climb

Amanze, A. and Truswell, D. (2023) 'The Blue Book to Recovery.' *Journal of Dementia Care, Equality, Diversity and Inclusion, Special Issue 31*, 5, 18–19.

BBC (2021) Reggae Memory Radio. www.bbc.co.uk/programmes/p09kll36

Doherty, J. (2021) Banjos (Dementia in Dub). https://youtu.be/CGz7iXrPLyI?si=4uioqKzpIpdlUMxL

Hawes, L. (2021) Amanze: Portrait of a Pirate. https://youtu.be/brGWHiEe-S0?si=8aDihcwjN5M_03un

Hitchmough, P. (2020) I'm Still Climbing Mountains. https://youtu.be/FD332QMCeXw?si=ezzFwH3zEDz7bqhG

My Dementia Life Matters (Talk Dementia with Ellie Robinson-Carter). https://ellierobinson-carter.com/The-Photobook-Project/My-Dementia-Life-Matters

CHAPTER 13

Social Prescribing of Creative Arts for Older People

Kate Parkin and Douglas Hunter

Introduction

This chapter introduces Equal Arts, a major Voluntary, Community and Social Enterprise (VCSE) creative arts organisation, and its work, and explores how older people get involved in its programmes via social prescribing (SP).

Following numerous attempts to engage link workers and promote our services, we wanted to understand why there were low rates of SP referrals to our programmes from statutory agencies. The opportunity to address these barriers arose when we became a VCSE provider with a local multi-agency prescribing consortium, Sunderland Social Prescribing Partnership (SSPP). The consortium, set up to test models of SP, aimed to raise public awareness and increase the number of people formally referred for a socially prescribed service in Sunderland.

During the SSPP programme, Equal Arts coordinated, delivered and evaluated a range of creative ageing programmes for older people and gained insights into local SP. In this chapter, we reflect on the organisational learning garnered through the project and our wider SP experiences, and share a list of actions to improve our visibility to partners and the public, advance local SP models and increase formal referrals to address health inequality.

Equal Arts

Equal Arts, founded in Gateshead in 1985, is a leading creative ageing charity based in North-East England with programmes across the country. The charity engages older people, including those living with dementia, in professionally led creative ageing activities designed to improve and maintain health and wellbeing. These provide stimulating and meaningful experiences that challenge stereotypes associated with ageing and contribute to more inclusive, cohesive and compassionate communities. Over four decades, Equal Arts has successfully collaborated with NHS trusts, local authority social services, and culture and voluntary sector partners, delivering creative ageing programmes that meet the psychosocial needs of vulnerable older people.

Older people usually join Equal Arts projects informally as self-referrals or are referred by their families searching for activities for their relatives. Local health and social care partners with whom we have strong links signpost patients and clients to us but we have found that very few referrals come via local SP.

Factors influencing low levels of referrals

The literature around SP in relation to the arts paints a complex picture with many different stakeholders, multiple mechanisms and, according to Polley *et al.* (2019), strong links to systems theory: '[a] model such as social prescribing is not a linear model, and, arguably subscribes more to systems theory and complexity theory in terms of understanding how a person at the centre of social prescribing actually benefits' (p.12). Stakeholders in SP may start in health, but the bulk of what SP needs to do requires collaboration between different kinds of community resources, including VCSE organisations. This calls for an infrastructure that works for patients because it's been co-designed by all the agencies who use it.

The hurdles to referrals include the relationships between link workers and arts professionals, and how the former's awareness of the ways arts organisations operate is predicated on how well the different parts of the system understand each other as touched on above (*ibid.*). How programmes are designed and communicated to patients and users of General Practitioner (GP) services and how the activities themselves are accessed are also important.

SP link-worker host organisations can also provide in-house services, which can be delivered by link-worker staff. Inevitably, signposting in-house is easier than understanding external provision, resulting in increased demand and the need for increased capacity within a service. Some link workers have also said they are only allowed to signpost into their own service.

Additional barriers include the short-term nature of some SP programmes and patient expectations, and the fear of psychosocial problems (Pescheny, Pappas and Randhawa 2018). Social anxiety and transport issues also play a part. In addition, Sumner *et al.* (2020) found that while people with lower levels of wellbeing may benefit most from participating in creativity, they may need more support to engage.

Whilst Equal Arts found shared practice with health professionals useful, other aspects of SP were frustrating. Some of the barriers to arts on prescription chime with SP research literature and clearly offer explanations for Equal Arts' experience (Clifford 2017, Crone *et al.* 2018, Pescheny *et al.* 2018, Polley *et al.* 2019, Aughterson, Baxter and Fancourt 2020, Baxter and Fancourt 2020, Fixsen *et al.* 2020).

Low referral numbers may also be related not only to GP and link-worker understanding of arts for health but also to patients' understanding of a social prescription and reluctance to engage in group activities, factors that may well be related to their psychological health, as well as family circumstances and social, economic or cultural factors (Skivington *et al.* 2018, Fixsen *et al.* 2020).

Our observation that local GPs seem to have low-level understanding of arts-for-health benefits is borne out in research. Although some professional healthcare and medical degree courses now include teaching arts for health and wellbeing, GPs and other health professionals more generally are unfamiliar with the benefits of non-medical interventions (Aughterson *et al.* 2020).

Successful referrals for creative arts rely on link workers having accurate information about local arts and cultural provision in order that they can support with emotional 'buy-in' (Fixsen *et al.* 2020), but maintaining up-to-date resource listings is a significant challenge.

A social prescribing case example

Since 2020, Equal Arts has been a member of the SSPP, along with the Sunderland GP Alliance, Sunderland Carers Centre and Groundwork, clearly demonstrating complexity and the need to work well with these different stakeholders. SSPP were one of 36 national projects awarded £50,000 by Arts Council England and the National Academy for Social Prescribing Thriving Communities Fund to test SP within a blended consortium approach (health, social, creative, sports and environmental) to improve wellbeing in areas of health inequality.

The SSPP partnership aimed to:

- build connections between the GP Alliance Social Prescribing Team, VCSE and creative organisations
- advocate and champion partner services that people can be referred to

- share information between partners/collaborative working
- develop quality principles to ensure confidence when referring carers to activities
- establish how learning from the 'Carers Pathway' pilot can support scale-up, supporting sustainability
- extend the partnership over the first year.

The purpose of the SSPP was to establish a city-wide strategic partnership to address health inequalities and support people affected by Coronavirus disease (COVID-19) by improving the range, quality and reach of SP activities in Sunderland. The 18-month project focused on supporting young carers, male carers and families caring for children and young people with special educational needs and disability, people living with dementia and their carers and older people with long-term health conditions and their carers.

The specific aims were to:

- enhance collaboration and networking between organisations
- strengthen the range and quality of 'healthy lives' activities offered in Sunderland
- enable Primary Care Network (PCN) SP teams to connect more people to more creative activities and to sustain this work over the duration of the project.

The roles of the GP Alliance in association with the PCN link workers and Sunderland Carers were to support the wider referral pathway into environmental, physical and creative activities provided by Groundwork and Equal Arts.

As a delivery partner, Equal Arts was commissioned to meet the health, wellbeing and social isolation needs of older people with dementia and their carers and older people with long-term health conditions and their carers, including those living with chronic obstructive pulmonary disease.

Working in south (Coalfields), west (Washington) and central Sunderland city wards, Equal Arts received 91 referrals: 45 referrals from SSPP consortium partners, 31 self-referrals and 15 recommendations from participants or family members.

Over 18 months Equal Arts delivered:

- 12 creative cafe 'drop ins' in Sunderland city centre and in the lounges of assisted living schemes; these sessions involved printmaking and ceramics and reached 28 people

- 12 doorstep creative activities consisting of singing and music on doorsteps, front gardens and streets, reaching at least 30 people
- 8 textile sessions at a care home in Sunderland Coalfields to support people living with dementia and their families, reaching 17 people
- 4 singing sessions at Easington Lane Community Centre to improve the breathing of people living with poor lung health
- 30 sessions of movement classes for people at risk of falls at leisure centres in West Sunderland; this Thriving Communities legacy project supported through Sunderland City Council Ageing Well Falls Prevention Programme and Covid-19 Health and Wellbeing Fund attracted 16 attendees over 7 months of weekly activity.

Results

Equal Arts collected and analysed statistical information about activities and qualitative feedback from participants to produce an evaluation that demonstrated health improvements for participants, including increased confidence, decreased low mood and improved physical health. Singing sessions not only helped lung capacity but also provided some participants with uplift in their mental wellbeing, which they, participants and family members reported as lasting long after the session had finished.

Similarly, participants' physical health, mood, social skills and physical confidence grew considerably over the six months of weekly activity and confidence-building at the Women's Strength and Balance sessions at Washington Leisure Centre. Participants progressed from light movement sessions to circus and trapeze sessions led by professional older people circus skills practitioners. Supported by two practitioners, participants would juggle, swing from ropes and hang from suspension slings. The evaluation, which gathered and analysed data from baseline interviews, specialist workshop observation, a focus group and interviews, showed improvements in social confidence for all and physical health improvements for the majority of participants.

As a result of the programme, four members of the group took up leisure centre membership for swimming. All 16 stayed after sessions for coffee and set up a WhatsApp social group to keep in touch.

> The social benefits of the project have brought sheer joy. A real sense of community spirit and engagement has grown within the group and individuals are supporting each other in their fitness journeys. (Member of the Strength and Balance sessions, Washington)

Discussion

To embed SP for arts and culture locally, there is much to do. We need arts and health networks that feed into and support each other in more joined up ways. We need to identify how best to share our SP offer in ways that are helpful to link workers. We need to understand what local health priorities we can address, for example, falls reduction, and understand what data is useful to capture and share. We need to understand which SP networks signpost to in-house services and which services want to work in partnership with external service providers. Sourcing longer-term funding is an ongoing challenge.

Our programme evaluation shows that the person- and group-centred outcomes resulted from sustained engagement between participants and skilled practitioners who build trusting relationships tailored to the needs of beneficiaries. They are threatened, however, by barriers discussed above, in particular how to overcome the problem of low take-up by way of referrals, which needs addressing from a whole-systems-thinking perspective (Fixsen *et al.* 2020).

After the end of the SSPP project, Equal Arts worked with partners and project participants to support access to creative arts and sustain the improvement in health of individual and groups who are interested in continuing to pursue these activities. We are currently working with 25 groups across Tyne and Wear.

Conclusion

Involvement in the SSPP project provided Equal Arts with greater insight into why, given our existing creative offer that accepts both informal and formal referrals at any point in time, we welcome few new members from SP link workers. It is clear that we need to improve our promotional information and improve our personal relationships with SP link workers on an individual and organisational level.

As a result of our SSPP and wider SP experience we shall:

- build on the inter-organisational relationships and the SP partnerships and continue to work with local agencies and organisations across the arts, health and social care sector
- continue to be represented on strategic groups, such as the integrated care system's ageing-well subgroup
- gain insight and understanding from arts organisations/voluntary sector providers in other parts of the UK that have developed, in conjunction with health and social care partners, an effective and

efficient referral pathway for SP that includes high-quality creative arts offers (Derbyshire Arts 2024)

- improve our promotional materials, which: (a) make the case for SP to use professionally trained and experienced creative arts practitioners, citing cost effectiveness studies of arts and culture on prescription which conclude that using creative arts/practitioners represents value for money; (b) recommend ways in which the local system of SP, including referral pathways, could continue to improve using best practice developed across the UK

- improve link workers' knowledge and understanding of the wider creative ageing sector. Currently, local link workers are not fully cognisant of the range of high-quality creative arts that Equal Arts provides and are therefore less likely to make a referral to us. We need to meet regularly to build mutual understanding and reciprocal relationships by sharing and exchanging information about our work.

LEARNING POINTS

- Consider our approaches to SP and build relationships with the partners who connect into local SP pathways to overcome barriers from multiple perspectives for the benefit of older people.

- Increase our dialogue with link workers, GP practices, public health, Health-works, adult social care and patients so we can collectively make more of a difference in addressing key health priorities and using evaluation methods that contribute to wider aggregated data sets.

- Advocate for longer-term funding that means SP arts programmes are sustainable and adequately resourced to address the health and wellbeing of older people, enhance the resilience of communities and significantly address health inequality.

References

Aughterson, H., Baxter, L. and Fancourt, D. (2020) 'Social prescribing for individuals with mental health problems: A qualitative study of barriers and enablers experienced by general practitioners.' *BMC Family Practice* 21, 194.

Baxter, L. and Fancourt, D. (2020) 'What are the barriers to, and enablers of, working with people with lived experience of mental illness amongst community and voluntary sector organisations? A qualitative study.' *PLoS One* 15, 7, e0235334.

Clifford, D. (2017) 'Charitable organisations, the Great Recession and the Age of Austerity: Longitudinal evidence for England and Wales.' *Journal of Social Policy* 46, 1, 1–30.

Crone, D. M., Sumner, R. C., Baker, C. M., Loughren, E. A., Hughes, S. and James, D. V. (2018) '"Artlift" arts-on-referral intervention in UK primary care: Updated findings from an ongoing observational study.' *The European Journal of Public Health* 28, 3, 404–409.

Derbyshire Arts (2024) *Social Prescribing Manifesto.* https://issuu.com/deborahartsderbyshire/docs/manifesto_pdf_combined

Fixsen, A., Seers, H., Polley, M. and Robins, J. (2020) 'Applying critical systems thinking to social prescribing: A relational model of stakeholder "buy-in".' *BMC Health Services Research* 20, 580.

Pescheny, J., Pappas, Y. and Randhawa, G. (2018) 'Facilitators and barriers of implementing and delivering social prescribing services: A systematic review.' *BMC Health Services Research* 18, 1, 86.

Polley, M., Whitehouse, J., Elnaschie, S. and Fixsen, A. (2019) *What Does Successful Social Prescribing Look Like: Mapping Meaningful Outcomes.* London: University of Westminster.

Skivington, K., Smith, M., Nai Rui, C., MacKenzie, M., Wyke, S. and Mercer, S. (2018) 'Delivering a primary care-based social prescribing initiative: A qualitative study of the benefits and challenges.' *British Journal of General Practice* 68, 672.

Sumner, R., Crone, D., Baker, C., Hughes, S., Loughren, E. and James, D. (2020) 'Factors associated with attendance, engagement and wellbeing change in an arts on prescription intervention.' *Journal of Public Health* 42, 1.

INFORMING, DEVELOPING and SUPPORTING

CHAPTER 14

Developing the Creative Health Workforce

Julia Puebla Fortier and Maria Pasiecznik Parsons

Introduction

This chapter examines the creative health workforce in the UK, identifying major drivers for the growth of a diverse workforce that consists of Creative Health Practitioners (CHPs), including Creative Arts Therapists (CATs) and Community Practitioners (CPs), whose training influences where and how they practise. Research highlights the complexity of the work, level of skill required, emotional rewards and psychologically exacting nature of relational practice, yet despite the existence of new postgraduate and undergraduate creative health degree courses, there is a significant shortfall in accessible and flexible training, professional development and psychosocial support options for this work. Creative Dementia Arts Network (CDAN) found course fees, costs and time commitment were major barriers for many practitioners and took these into account in developing FLOURISH, a practice-learning course in creative arts and dementia. The Culture, Health and Wellbeing Alliance (CHWA), National Centre for Creative Health (NCCH), national arts councils, Baring Foundation and NHS are continuing to promote creative health workforce development and increase practitioner support. Stakeholder collaboration is important in supporting the development of entry-level preparation and a lifelong learning pathway to ensure the calibre of the workforce.

Background

The growth of the creative health workforce signals increased recognition of the health and wellbeing benefits of participatory arts and culture for adults and older people amongst arts, health, social care and housing with care organisations. At the same time, health and social care policies are evolving in response to the support needs of an ageing population with age-related disability and dementia. Creative health advocates and organisations are now working more closely with the NHS as it reconfigures its workforce to facilitate the shift of healthcare from acute settings into primary care and communities through Integrated Care Boards, which plan services for improving health, reducing inequalities in local populations and supporting personalised care.

Demand for a trained creative health workforce is also being driven by the systematic implementation of social prescribing (SP) in the UK, including the development of arts and culture SP to meet psychological and social needs. The National Academy for Social Prescribing (NASP) is cataloguing research that shows positive outcomes for SP (for example, Mughal *et al.* 2022), although the SP system does not yet have the capacity to fully respond to NHS waiting lists for complex health interventions. Some studies identify problems in referral systems and a lack of communication between the third sector and health care (both flagged in Chapter 13) and others highlight concerns about safeguarding participants and practitioners given a lack of ethical guidelines for arts and health practice (Wilson *et al.* 2016, Brown, Tierney and Turk 2019, Calderon 2021, Bungay, Jensen and Holt 2023).

The creative health workforce

Creative health activities in the UK may be delivered by artists, community volunteers or Allied Health Professionals; indeed, anyone with an interest in creative activities for health or wellbeing can deliver creative health activities (Fortier 2023). CHPs therefore have a wide range of professional training and qualifications.

The Health Care and Professions Council (HCPC) approves postgraduate creative arts therapy courses, registers CATs, music therapists and drama therapists and ensures members adhere to professional standards of conduct, performance, ethics, proficiency and continuing professional development. The Association for Dance and Movement Psychotherapy (ADMP) is a professional organisation with the same regulatory responsibilities for dance and movement psychotherapists. Clinical supervision is a mandatory practice requirement for all registered CATs. CATs work mainly in clinical healthcare settings and for large care home providers, although a growing number work in community settings. Regular clinical supervision is provided by the NHS or other employers.

CHPs have wider educational backgrounds ranging from graduate qualifications in arts, music, dance, drama, etc. to being self-taught. Some of those working with older adults will have undertaken training in using their art form for working with this population, but most learn by experience, sometimes in residence in care homes (Algar-Skaife, Caulfield and Woods 2017). The majority of practitioners work in the community, with arts organisations, with arts and cultural venues and in social care and housing with care settings. A large group are independent practitioners, and many are self-employed and work as freelancers on short-term projects, managing precarious work portfolios. Employers of practitioners with full-time or permanent part-time contracts sometimes provide supervision. The work of CHPs is not regulated by a professional body responsible for standards, so they have no professional or ethical obligation to engage in continuous professional development or in practice supervision. Regular paid-for supervision and other psychosocial practice support is very far from being the norm for the creative health workforce (Naismith 2019, Fortier and Massey-Chase 2024) as discussed in Chapter 15.

Information about the size of the creative health workforce is limited although the Culture, Health and Wellbeing Alliance (CHWA) has estimated that it is 10,000. This figure is not disaggregated by type of role, mode of employment or specialism, such as people living with dementia (which is a fast-growing field given an ageing population and increasing prevalence of dementia).

Lack of current data about the creative health sector and its workforce was the impetus for *Creative Health: UK State of the Sector Survey* (Tang 2024). Despite a low response rate, results from CHPs and managers provide a snapshot of who works in the creative health sector, their geographic location, art form, motivation for work, work settings, earnings, training and professional development and whether they evaluate their work and future prospects for the sector. Tang (2024 p.12) concludes that 'it would seem that creative health is becoming more widely accepted and integrated into current healthcare systems' but highlights freelancers' pay, training and development needs as requiring action by the sector.

The workforce and training needs

Recent research on the experiences of 43 arts, health and wellbeing facilitators (practitioners) in England documents how frequently artists work with participants living with challenging health conditions or social situations (Fortier 2023). These artists describe their main tasks as facilitating creativity, encouraging social engagement and making space for expression and emotion. They also spoke about the emotional demands of the practice and challenges that can include managing medical and psychological crises, behavioural issues and disclosures of abuse and trauma.

These challenges are intensified for some facilitators, who feel unsure about the parameters of their role and responsibilities, their training and experience or the level of support they receive. Facilitators report using a variety of strategies to manage this complexity, including working with participant carers and co-facilitators, conveying empathy while setting emotional boundaries and seeking out support through self-care, supervision and peer relationships. Those new to the work often struggle with self-confidence, and those with lived experience use their knowledge and skills to manage provocative situations but may also feel vulnerable at times. For unskilled and/or unsupported artists, these challenges could also compromise the benefits of the intervention or the safety of participants. Many facilitators, however, said they reflect on and process their experiences from challenging encounters so that they become lessons and tools for future work (Fortier 2023).

A recent literature review of arts on prescription identifies a need for more defined training and qualifications for artists working in this context given they have to account for the complex needs of participants, manage the social aspects of creative activity and attend to a duty of care in SP referrals (Bungay *et al.* 2023). In the Fortier study (2023), many experienced facilitators pursued a range of courses and personal study on different topics for their work, including specialised content related to the conditions of people they worked with (Fortier 2023). Others said they'd had no induction or training prior to their first experiences of working with people with complex needs and that this sometimes negatively impacted on their confidence and ability to respond appropriately in challenging circumstances. Even experienced facilitators with some training said they found that the disclosure of abuse or manifestations of serious mental health problems during sessions could be disorienting and disturbing – for them and for other participants.

On-the-job experience was most often cited as a key learning pathway: 'While several facilitators described how instinct guides their practice and responses, others said they would value a more structured practice framework or accreditation process to guide their practice and signal competencies and quality' (Fortier 2023 p.121). Currently, the lack of professional training and competency requirements means that facilitators may or may not pursue training on topics that might help them develop the relevant preparatory knowledge and skills to work with people with challenging or complex needs. This is of concern, given increasing anecdotal and emerging qualitative evidence of significant levels of burnout, exhaustion and vicarious trauma across the workforce, with only intermittent access to supervision, support and ethical guidance (Shorter, McCann and McIlherron 2018, Fortier and Massey-Chase 2024).

Professional training and continuing professional development

Historically, the rationale for formal training for arts and health work speaks to having the knowledge and skills to adequately respond to vulnerable individuals and their complex needs (Moss 2016). Moss and O'Neill (2009) note that, without such preparation, 'it is possible that the quality of intervention by artists could vary, and at times this might pose a risk to patients through breach of confidentiality or unawareness of emotional supports needed for patients engaging in arts activities' (p.4). They identified a set of core themes central for any proposed courses for arts and health, including:

> …ethics; hospital and healthcare settings environment; patient-/client-centred care; self-awareness and motivation; value of arts and health/best practice; therapy; overview of nature of disease; facilitation/group work skills; the nature of collaborative practice; research skills; language and communication skills; project planning and development skills; and an overview of arts and health. Placements and mentors were identified as crucial to successful implementation of such courses. (*ibid.* p.4)

While many freelance practitioners have cited cost and time as barriers to pursuing formal study in creative health, several universities have launched postgraduate creative health courses, including the Creative Health MASc (Master of Arts and Sciences) at University College London, the MA in Arts, Health and Wellbeing at Plymouth Marjon University and the MA in Arts Practice (Arts Health and Wellbeing) at the University of South Wales. Increasing numbers of courses are being offered at undergraduate level, such as the BA (Hons) in Therapeutic Practice at the City of Bristol College, accredited by Bath Spa University, and the Creative Expressive Arts, Health and Wellbeing BA (Hons) at the University of Derby. Community-based training programmes of varying lengths are also being offered in cities around the UK.

Outside the creative arts therapy professions, no UK arts, higher education, adult training or accrediting body has undertaken standard-setting work on the knowledge, skills and competencies needed by artists to deliver non-clinical creative health programmes. As a result, there is no system of entry-level qualification or continuous professional development that is linked to a defined set of competencies. There is still ongoing debate about the demarcation between clinical and non-clinical creative health practice that complicates this issue. It may be useful to view the creative health workforce on a continuum of practice and competencies. First proposed by Moss in 2016 and further developed in the USA, Betts and Huet propose a framework for mapping and guiding workforce development and training in creative health, which identifies the range of settings, skills and intentions that characterise and differentiate clinical situated arts therapies from community arts practice (Betts and Huet 2023 p.6). These distinctions in terms of training and practice roles have been explored and evolved over time (Dileo and Bradt 2009, Van Lith and Spooner 2018).

High-quality creative health practice encompasses a broad range of practice approaches, settings and participant groups, each requiring different knowledge and skills, which makes the task of developing a comprehensive framework for education and training challenging. However, the Creative Health Quality Framework offers practitioners, commissioners and providers eight detailed principles of good practice and guidance to design, deliver or commission creative health programmes (Hume and Willis 2023).

Creative Practitioners working with people living with dementia

Much of this narrative resonates with the training and professional development experience of CDAN, a small arts charity focused on training and support for creative arts practitioners who work with people living with dementia. It is difficult to estimate the size of this workforce, but all CHPs working with older people are likely to engage with people living with the condition given that 1 in 11 people aged 65 years and over are living with dementia.

The development of FLOURISH, CDAN's creative arts and dementia practice learning course, drew on evaluation data about training needs collected during CDAN projects, programmes, conferences and training courses between 2011 and 2019 (n = 1247). Results showed that the creative arts and dementia workforce is composed of small to medium arts organisations and independent creative arts and health practitioners, of whom an estimated 70% are self-employed and work on short-term contracts (Pasiecznik Parsons 2019). Respondents, particularly freelancers, generally self-fund their training and continuing professional development (CPD); most identified affordability as a major deterrent, followed by lack of local availability and course flexibility. They also highlighted the absence of practice learning opportunities on courses.

There is no education training and professional development pathway for CHPs wishing to work with people living with dementia, and a rapid search of all UK creative arts and dementia education, training and professional development courses identified a plethora of different opportunities, including postgraduate and undergraduate modules courses, short courses and workshops offered by arts organisations, freelance practitioners and universities.

Online resources include a self-directed arts and dementia course available on FutureLearn and downloadable practice guidance materials and toolkits (*ibid.*). A rapid mapping review of training provision for artists working in care homes reinforced CDAN's view that current training and professional development resources are of variable quality (Allen 2018). Few are kite-marked, although some are user-rated.

CDAN's FLOURISH course was designed to meet the needs of both early career creative arts practitioners and those seeking to update practice. FLOURISH initially comprised a day's course, plus self-study, mentoring, reflective practice sessions and a supervised practice placement of eight hours in an arts or care setting. Face-to-face interactive teaching and learning in a group of 14 learners was led by a course leader with considerable experience of dementia care practice, training and running arts and dementia projects. All teaching materials were printed and distributed. Following evaluation of the pilot, the taught course was extended to two days for the second student cohort. Students positively evaluated FLOURISH, rating the practice learning component particularly highly. The pilot included a day event that aimed to help those completing FLOURISH (and was open to other CHPs) who wanted to establish themselves as independent practitioners. Numbers of attendees and very positive evaluation signals this as a professional development need.

Coordination and collaboration as the way forward

Workforce development is being addressed by major creative health stake-holders including CHWA, NCCH, arts councils in England, Wales, Scotland and Northern Ireland and the Baring Foundation. Sector support organisations in Wales and Ireland are developing training and guidance on working conditions for CHPs, and in England, there are efforts underway to identify core competencies for CHPs. Local creative health organisations are also piloting training initiatives. Creative health policy and programmes are one of the priorities of Arts Council England (ACE), whose *Creative Health & Wellbeing Plan* (ACE 2022) includes support for creative practitioner skills development. NHS England is considering the training needs for future arts, drama and music therapy workforce needs (Moula 2023). The USA has developed a core curriculum for arts and health practice that is the basis for an emerging voluntary certification programme (Wikoff *et al.* 2021), which might well offer a model for other countries.

While many CHPs assert the primacy of their artist identity, research and practice shows that they draw on multiple skills, knowledge and experiences to work with different art forms and participants with varying health conditions in many different settings. By collaborating with funders, delivery partners and other stakeholders, leaders in the creative health field can support better practitioner experiences and practices by recognising and responding to the complexity, demands and emotional impact of working with individuals with challenging conditions or situations. They can address the ambiguity of the role and responsibilities by developing practice guidance for facilitators, identifying essential competencies for working with challenging conditions and creating a professional development pathway based on tacit and explicit practice knowledge, skills development and mentored, experience-based learning. As the evidence base for creative health grows and adoption broadens across health and social care, the demand for practitioners who can deliver safe and effective programmes will increase.

ACE has proposed supporting skills-development activities, including collaborating with the NHS to develop training resources for creative and cultural workers. Commissioners, practitioners and participants will benefit from consistent guidance and professional structures that more clearly define the preparation, role, responsibilities and working conditions for creative health practice aligned with quality standards. The future growth of creative health depends on the calibre of its workforce, hence the need for key stakeholders to collaborate on a systematic approach to making training, professional development and support opportunities available throughout the creative health practice trajectory.

LEARNING POINTS

- Engaging people living with dementia in creative arts can help to meet their psychological and social needs and those of their carers.

- Research highlights not only the rewards of the work but also the emotional demands of the practice and challenges, including managing medical and psychological crises, behavioural issues and disclosures of abuse and trauma.

- Many CHPs learn by experience, given the dearth of training and professional development opportunities.

- Training and professional development, and practitioner support initiatives by major stakeholders, need to be progressed in order to provide a workforce fit for a more integrated health and social care service focused on meeting social need at primary and community level.

References

Algar-Skaife, K., Caulfield, M. and Woods, B. (2017) *cARTrefu: Creating Artists in Residents. A National Arts in Care Homes Participatory and Mentoring Programme: Evaluation Report 2015–2017*. Cardiff: Age Cymru. www.agecymru.wales/siteassets/documents/cartrefu/age-cymru-english---evaluation-report.pdf

Allen, P. (2018) *Arts in Care Homes*. London: The Baring Foundation. https://baringfoundation.org.uk/resource/arts-in-care-homes-a-rapid-mapping-of-training-provision

Arts Council England (2022) *Creative Health and Wellbeing*. Manchester: Arts Council England. www.artscouncil.org.uk/developing-creativity-and-culture/health-and-wellbeing/creative-health-wellbeing

Betts, D. and Huet, V. (2023) *Bridging the Creative Arts Therapies and Arts for Health*. London: Jessica Kingsley Publishers.

Brown, R, Tierney, S. and Turk, A. (2019) The ethics of social prescribing: An overview. NIHR School for Primary Care Research. www.spcr.nihr.ac.uk/news/blog/the-ethics-of-social-prescribing-an-overview

Bungay, H., Jensen, A. and Holt, N. (2023) 'Critical perspectives on Arts on Prescription.' *Perspectives in Public Health* 144, 6, 363–368.

Calderón-Larrañaga, S., Milner, Y., Clinch, M., Greenhalgh, T. and Finer, S. (2021) 'Tensions and opportunities in social prescribing. Developing a framework to facilitate its implementation and evaluation in primary care: a realist review.' *British Journal of General Practice Open 5*, 3.

Dileo, C. and Bradt, J. (2009) 'On creating the discipline, profession, and evidence in the field of arts and healthcare.' *Arts Health 1*, 2, 168–182.

Fortier, J. P. (2023) 'Navigating Ambiguity and Boundaries: The Experiences of Arts, Health and Wellbeing Facilitators Working with Individuals with Challenging Conditions or Situations.' Doctoral thesis. London: London School of Hygiene and Tropical Medicine. https://doi.org/10.17037/PUBS.04671753

Fortier, J. and Massey-Chase, K. (2024) *Keeping Safe: A Review of Psychosocial and Wellbeing Support Options for Creative Practitioners Working with Challenging Conditions and Circumstances*. Manchester: Arts Council England.

Hume, V. and Willis, J. (2023) Creative Health Quality Framework. Culture, Health and Wellbeing Alliance. www.culturehealthandwellbeing.org.uk/resources/creative-health-quality-framework

Moss, H. (2016) 'Arts and health: A new paradigm.' *Voices: A World Forum for Music Therapy 16*, 3. https://voices.no/index.php/voices/article/view/2301

Moss, H. and O'Neill, D. (2009) 'What training do artists need to work in healthcare settings?' *Medical Humanities 35*, 2, 101–105.

Moula, Z. (2023) *Identifying Priorities in Future Workforce of Art, Drama, and Music Therapy, and Promoting Examples of Good Practice in Postgraduate Training Programmes across the UK*. Developed with the British Association of Dramatherapists (BADth), British Association for Music Therapy (BAMT) and British Association of Art Therapists (BAAT). Leeds: NHS England.

Mughal, R., Polley, M., Sabey, A. and Chatterjee, H. J. (2022) *How Arts, Heritage and Culture can Support Health and Wellbeing through Social Prescribing*. London: National Association of Social Prescribing.

Naismith, N. (2019) Artists practising well. Aberdeen: Robert Gordon University. https://doi.org/10.48526/rgu-wt-235847

Pasiecznik Parsons, M. (2019) *The Training Needs of Creative Arts, Health and Wellbeing Practitioners Working with People Living with Dementia*. Oxford: Creative Dementia Arts Network (Unpublished).

Shorter, G. W., McCann, S. and McIlherron, L. (2018) *Changing Arts and Minds: A Survey of Health and Wellbeing in the Creative Sector*. Belfast: Inspire.

Tang, J. (2024) *Creative Health: UK State of the Sector Survey*. Barnsley: Culture, Health and Wellbeing Alliance.

Van Lith, T. and Spooner, H. (2018) 'Art therapy and arts in health: Identifying shared values but different goals using a framework analysis.' *Art Therapy* 35, 2, 88–93.

Wikoff, N., de Boer, C., Speiser, V. M., Sims, E. *et al.* (2021) *Core Curriculum for Arts in Health Professionals.* Houston, TX: National Organization of Arts in Health.

Wilson, C., Bungay, H., Munn-Giddings, C. and Boyce, M. (2016) 'Healthcare professionals' perceptions of the value and impact of the arts in healthcare settings: A critical review of the literature.' *International Journal of Nursing Studies* 56, 90–101.

CHAPTER 15

Support for Creative Practitioners

Nicola Naismith

Introduction

This chapter makes the case for Creative Practitioners (CPs) in arts and health to be better supported in their rewarding, but often challenging, work, particularly when working with people living with dementia and their professional and familial carers. It identifies the reasons why support is often not available and explores the obstacles to and consequences of not getting adequate support, before describing the different kinds of support available. It offers the idea of a menu approach to support, highlighting the importance of choice in both support and reflection methods, which when combined, can be used by CPs to expand and develop practice.

This chapter is important for commissioners of arts and dementia work, Creative Arts Therapists (CATs) and CPs. Unlike CATs, whose conditions of service include regular supervision with a qualified clinical supervisor (see Chapter 18), CPs' support needs remain largely unmet. This chapter will lead to a better understanding of the work structures and support needs of CPs, and through this, will facilitate better-informed dialogue, collaboration and mutual support between these distinct but connected groups of workers.

Issues pertaining to Creative Practitioner support
Asking for help, learning from other professions and the culture of coping

When presenting my first research study into the support needs of CPs working in arts in health contexts (Naismith 2019), an audience question arose: how do we get over the idea that asking for help is a sign of weakness? At the time, my response was that asking for help needs to be seen as a sign of strength and professionalism, as this work can give rise to a combination of feelings that are at times likely – on the balance of probability alone – to be challenging in nature.

Since then, my research has developed to explore the ways in which other people-orientated professions (for example, nursing and teaching) embed reflective practice and supervision into their training and work practices, which enables work-based experiences to be processed and supports continuing professional development (CPD). CPs working in participatory arts may come into arts and dementia work via art-form-specific training, or be self-taught, and so may have few opportunities to experience what support is, why it is needed and what forms it takes. Additionally, career development in the creative arts for CPs is often built on 'making do' and adapting, as opportunities and funding are hard to secure. This 'making do' can lead to a reluctance to identify as being *'in need'*, which often prevents CPs from asking for or accessing support with processing work-based experiences (Naismith 2021 p.33). Furthermore, if the support being offered is provided by the commissioning organisation, complexities around appearing needy in a potentially economically competitive environment can contribute to what I describe as a *culture of coping (ibid.* p.33). CPs may then seek to mask difficulties in order to 'steady the ship', a practice that can be seen in the wider arts sector (Freelancers Make Theatre Work 2021 p.18).

Feelings of isolation

CPs working with people living with dementia primarily work in health and social care settings, and with community arts organisations and arts venues. They are usually independent freelancers who work alongside volunteers and employed staff, and their work is often sessional and/or short-term, involving time-limited interactions with participants. Due to the way their work is commissioned, where it is located and the nature of arts in health work (which may not be fully understood by employed staff), these practitioners occupy a distinctly peripheral and isolated space in many organisations that contract them (Collard-Stokes and Irons 2022).

This situation may not be inherently problematic, but CPs may witness events and experience practice challenges for which they have not been fully trained, and without support from commissioners and wider participatory arts structures, these experiences can remain unprocessed. These elements combined can lead to feelings of isolation (Baxter and Fancourt 2020, Collard-Stokes and Irons 2022, O'Connor 2022), which can be exacerbated further through a work culture that normalises coping (Naismith 2021 p.33). The interconnected challenges experienced by CPs include:

- the isolation and marginalisation of freelancers whose work is largely periodic and temporary
- the systemic inequalities central to the arts and culture sector
- the reliance on short-term funding, for which there is intense competition between organisations and subsequently between freelance practitioners for any project offered
- inadequate access to support within commissioning organisations.

Relational aspects of participatory arts, ethical dilemmas and lived experience

The relational aspects of participatory arts are central to, but often at odds with, funding structures, which can limit the duration of projects, interrupt the collaborative process and lead to unsatisfactory endings (Belfiore 2022). Working creatively with others brings joy, purpose, difficulty and challenge; a complex web of feelings that sit alongside the ethical dilemmas inherent within participatory arts work (Goldbard and Matarasso 2021).

CPs' own wider lived experiences need consideration; for example, they may have a friend or family member living with dementia or another neurological condition, or there may be an absence of experience if they have never visited a care home or met anyone with a dementia diagnosis. Hatton (2021) traces her own history of contact with care homes, naming feelings which lead to the identification of assumptions – *what we think to be true* – and can be ill-informed, unrealistic and unhelpful to both CPs and the people they work with (Naismith 2021 p.16). Naming and reflecting upon these autobiographical beliefs related to a particular space or group of people encourages critical thinking and challenges hegemonic assumptions (Brookfield 1998 p.197, Bolton and Delderfield 2018 p.54).

Consequences of a lack of support

By acknowledging the barriers around asking for help in an established culture of coping, the challenges of working outside of existing support structures and the isolation that comes with freelance work, a complex picture emerges. Problematic funding structures and individual lived experience further contribute to the complexity: without support activities and reflective spaces, there is a real risk of overwhelm, compassion fatigue, psychological ill health, vicarious trauma and/or burnout (Naismith 2021, O'Connor 2022). It is both logical and appropriate for CPs' work-based experiences to be processed within a framework that is at least in part attached to the work environment. Failure to do so places the emphasis on the individual CP to self-resource, which is an unsustainable and unethical burden.

Meeting Creative Practitioner support needs
Creating an inclusive culture of support

This section highlights the importance of reflection in support for CPs, but what follows can be expanded to include any care workers, family members, activity coordinators and health staff involved in a project or session. Viewing support and reflection as encompassing activities that welcome multiple viewpoints contributes to a greater sense of shared learning and aids the development of practice (Bassot 2016 pp.108–109).

The differences between self-care and support

Before detailing support types and methods, it is useful to differentiate between self-care and support, as the terms are often used interchangeably. The origins of self-care can be found in the work of activist and writer Audre Lorde (1988), but the term has since been appropriated and commercialised into packages of resilience, wellness and self-improvement that can be purchased (The Care Collective 2020, Dowling 2021). Some of these iterations of self-care can be life affirming – holidays, activities with friends or pursuing hobbies – but they require time and financial resources, which are not always available to CPs (Collard-Stokes and Irons 2022, Naismith 2021). These activities alone cannot be an antidote to an unhealthy work culture or a lack of fair pay, and nor can they unpick a worrying concern or answer a persistent question. What good-quality support offers – in its myriad forms – is the opportunity to identify, reflect and process work-based experiences and feelings, so as to enable the individual practitioner to learn and develop their practice, whilst also contributing to the overall development of the field.

Instrumental support

Support has two constituent parts – instrumental and affective – which have a symbiotic relationship. The first – instrumental support – is concerned with contracts, pay, induction and orienteering sessions, team introductions, points of contact and discussions about access needs. These are all best attended to well before the commencement of the work, as doing so lays solid foundations for practice. A good practice example is offered in the Arts in Care Homes project, a Luminate training initiative that highlights the importance of induction and full-day visits, with artists spending time with both care staff and residents ahead of sessions. Both CPs and care staff reflected on how beneficial this preparation was, with care staff reporting an increased level of understanding about the activities the artists would be facilitating and the support they might need (Research Scotland 2022 p.16).

Affective support

Affective support is focused on processing the thoughts, feelings and attitudes that arise before, during and after a work session. Quite often, clinical supervision, a practice requirement for CATs, is held up as the gold standard of support, and indeed, it is increasingly available for CPs (see Chapter 18). However, other types of support can meet practitioners' needs, including action learning sets, coaching, creative practice, embodied practices, mentoring and reverse mentoring, peer learning spaces, research, team meetings, training and writing (for more information about each of these see Naismith 2021 pp.17–25).

Adopting a menu approach to affective support

Offering CPs different methods and approaches to affective support enables them to select a combination which can include those that they have prior experience of, and/or others that they are curious about, to create their own individual support menu. Congruence with CPs' needs and preferences increases the likelihood of their effectiveness. Some support activities can be self-organised, for instance a reflective journal that records events, feelings and action points, or a conversation with a peer. Other activities that are designed and delivered by organisations, and require paid time to attend, include externally facilitated peer groups and action learning sets. Additionally, participating in seminar and conference events will enable CPs to access and contribute to developmental practice and research discussions.

Support is going to look different for everyone and is dependent on the nature, duration and complexity of the work being undertaken and the individual needs of CPs. It is also likely to change over time: working with a more experienced mentor may give way to prioritising a regular peer-to-peer conversation or a facilitated reflective practice group (Naismith 2022). In order to design an individual support menu, CPs first need to have access to different types of support and then experiment with using them. A combination of online and in-person support facilitates greater inclusion for CPs who live in rural areas, have caring responsibilities and/or face economic barriers that may prevent travel away from home (Naismith 2021 p.25).

The role of reflection in support

Reflection is at the centre of affective support and can be described as in-depth focused attention (Bolton and Delderfield 2018 p.xxii), which leads to practice development through a greater understanding and awareness of *what* is happening and *why*. Reflective practice counters a culture of coping by bringing experiences out into the open, facilitating greater empathy between

CPs, and by extension, the participants they work with (*ibid.* p.2). Reflecting is a core component of quality practice and is further described in Chapter 2.

One of the most well-known reflective models is that of Schön (1992), which focuses on *reflection in action* – which takes place in the process of action – and *reflection on action* – which happens after a session or interaction. Both are useful ways to frame experience, but it is also helpful to include *reflection before action* (Edwards 2017), which offers opportunities for CPs to notice the conditions around them, as well as their own thoughts and feelings, to establish what they need from themselves and to identify the requests they need to make before the work happens.

Beyond Schön, there are numerous other reflective practice models and frameworks – some originally developed for nursing and education contexts – each with a different emphasis and purpose that can be adapted and applied to the work CPs undertake. Brookfield (2017), Gibbs (1998), Jasper (2013), Kolb (1984) and Rolfe, Freshwater and Jasper (2001) all offer different ways to harness the learning potential from practice and professional activities. An online search for any of these will result in a range of written descriptions, diagrammatic representations and video explanations, with university resources being particularly helpful (see University of Hull n.d.). These models are best experimented with, and over time, a preference or preferences usually emerge. They can also be adapted, combined and extended, and used for both individual and peer-group reflection to support practice development and enquiry.

Reflective practice framework models foreground critical thinking, encouraging us to go beyond a surface appraisal and supporting deeper dives into practice experiences and questions that do not have a single *answer* or issues that are not easy to *solve*. By using reflection to prioritise questions, issues or areas for change, *incremental next steps* can be identified, which in turn supports the sustainability of practice development. Reflection is essentially an ongoing process: if reflective discussion only takes place at the end of a project, and only then to facilitate the completion of a funding evaluation report, vital opportunities to reflect during the process are missed and may leave CPs with unexplored complex questions and concerns over an extended period of time. Much like the type of support activities CPs choose, the frequency of reflection also needs to fit in with their working lives. A combination of regular reflection before, during and after sessions or project delivery is likely to be useful, with deeper dives into practice being periodically timetabled.

Support in relation to structural challenges

Support activities and reflective practice are also useful when considering structural issues within arts in health and the wider cultural sector. It remains the case that access is required to economic, social and cultural resources in order to develop a career in the cultural sector (Brook, O'Brien and Taylor 2020). Furthermore, research that explored the impact of the COVID-19 pandemic on freelance and self-employed arts workers found that cancelled work and reduced hours resulted in high levels of stress and concern (Florisson *et al.* 2021). Where work was retained, there was a need to quickly reinvent creative activities for online or postal working (Naismith 2020). The insufficient care for families supporting relatives at home – combined with the challenges staff face around pay, training and time in care home settings (Dowling 2021) – will be witnessed by CPs. These and other structural issues are 'in the field' for many CPs, even before any creative work with participants takes place.

Many of these structural issues are beyond the reach of individual problem solving, but by exploring and acknowledging where particular challenges are located, situations can be viewed more holistically and individuals steered away from an aggravated sense of personal responsibility. Support and reflective activities have a key part to play in identifying actions or next steps, highlighting what sits with the individual and their practice or a wider landscape of practice, and what pertains to wider structures in arts in health – and beyond (Naismith 2021 p.16).

Identifying and celebrating successes

Much of this chapter has been focused on the challenging issues that CPs may face, both in the set-up of the work and in practice. However, it is also important to observe and acknowledge when practice is going well – when sessions/projects feel positive, both for practitioner and participants, and when feedback is encouraging. Taking time to notice this – individually and/or collectively – helps to identify what conditions were in place, which in turn helps to build incremental changes in practice (Brookfield 2017 pp.150–151). Reflective practice can most certainly be used in the service of exploring challenges, but equally, it can be used to identify, highlight and celebrate where things are working. Sharing a full range of experiences within supportive structures is essential in helping to build a robust community of practice within creative arts and dementia.

Conclusion

This chapter explored some of the issues pertaining to support for practitioners, in particular CPs: their freelance status, the prevalence of short-term and sessional employment and the lack of organisational support leading to feelings of isolation. The complexity of the work undertaken by CPs – and the risks involved in not providing support – is illustrated by the barriers around asking for help and the associated risk of appearing needy in a culture of coping; and the differences between self-care and support, instrumental and affective support are key. Regular access to inclusive, supportive and reflective practices are essential, as they enable CPs to process and identify insights from their work-based experiences – both challenging and celebratory. From this supported position, CPs will be better placed to undertake arts and dementia work and to contribute to wider practice and sector developments.

LEARNING POINTS

It is essential that commissioners and CATs support CPs to:

- identify their support needs
- understand the support options available
- access a range of support and reflective practice activities
- communicate the challenges and successes of practice.

References

Bassot, B. (2016) *The Reflective Practice Guide: An Interdisciplinary Approach to Critical Reflection.* Abingdon: Routledge.

Baxter, L. and Fancourt, D. (2020) 'What are the barriers to, and enablers of, working with people with lived experience of mental illness amongst community and voluntary sector organisations? A qualitative study.' *PLoS ONE 15,* 7, e0235334.

Belfiore, E. (2022) 'Who cares? At what price? The hidden costs of socially engaged arts labour and the moral failure of cultural policy.' *European Journal of Cultural Studies 25,* 1, 61–78.

Bolton, G. and Delderfield, R. (2018) *Reflective Practice: Writing and Professional Development.* London: Sage.

Brook, O., O'Brien D. and Taylor, M. (2020) *Culture Is Bad for You: Inequality in the Cultural and Creative Industries.* Manchester: Manchester University Press.

Brookfield, S. (1998) 'Critically reflective practice.' *The Journal of Continuing Education in the Health Professions 18,* 197–205.

Brookfield, S. (2017) *Becoming a Critically Reflective Teacher.* 2nd edition. San Francisco, CA: Jossey-Bass.

Collard-Stokes, G. and Irons, J. (2022) 'Artist wellbeing: Exploring the experiences of dance artists delivering community health and wellbeing initiatives.' *Research in Dance Education 23,* 1, 60–74.

Dowling, E. (2021) *The Care Crisis: What Caused It and How Can We End It?* London: Verso.

Edwards, S. (2017) 'Reflecting differently. New dimensions: Reflection-before-action and reflection-beyond-action.' *International Practice Development Journal 7,* 1, 2.

Florisson, R., O'Brien, D., Taylor, M., McAndrew, S. and Feder, T. (2021) The impact of Covid-19 on jobs in the cultural sector – part 3. www.culturehive.co.uk/CVIresources/the-impact-of-covid-19-on-jobs-in-the-cultural-sector-part-3

Freelancers Make Theatre Work (2021) *The Big Freelancer Report 2021*. https://freelancersmaketheatrework.com/wp-content/uploads/2021/03/The-Big-Freelancer-Report.pdf

Goldbard, A. and Matarasso, F. (2021) *Ethics and Participatory Art: Calouste Gulbenkian Foundation*. https://content.gulbenkian.pt/wp-content/uploads/2021/05/05120439/2021_AC_Ethics-and-Participatory-Art.pdf

Gibbs, G. (1988) *Learning by Doing, A Guide to Teaching and Learning*. Oxford Centre for Staff and Learning Development, Oxford: Oxford Brookes University. https://thoughtsmostlyaboutlearning.wordpress.com/wp-content/uploads/2015/12/learning-by-doing-graham-gibbs.pdf

Hatton, N. (2021) *Performance and Dementia: A Cultural Response to Care*. Zurich: Palgrave Macmillan.

Jasper, M. (2013) *Beginning Reflective Practice*. 2nd edition. Andover: Cengage Learning.

Kolb, D. A. (1984) *Experiential Learning: Experience as the Source of Learning and Development*. Englewood Cliffs, NJ: Prentice Hall.

Lorde, A. (1988) *A Burst of Light and Other Essays*. New York: Ixia Press.

Naismith, N. (2019) *Artists Practising Well*. Aberdeen: Robert Gordon University.

Naismith, N. (2020) *Adapting/Translating/Re-Inventing: Reflections on the Cultural Institute 'Beyond Measure' Twitter Chat*. https://static1.squarespace.com/static/5cd14cb8e8ba448eb9b87f6e/t/61d84a8935f6f71c78427969/1641564810980/NicolaNaismith_BeyondMeasure_August2020.pdf

Naismith, N. (2021) *Practising Well: Conversations and Support Menu*. Aberdeen: Robert Gordon University.

Naismith, N. (2022) *Flourishing Lives Reflective Practice Groups Evaluation Report*. https://flourishinglives.org/flourishing-lives-reflective-practice-groups-report

O'Connor, A. (2022) 'The work hurts.' *Journal of Applied Arts & Health* 13, 2, 153–166.

Research Scotland (2022) *Evaluation of the Arts in Care Project*. Research Scotland. https://luminatescotland.org/wp-content/uploads/2023/03/Arts-in-Care-Final-Report-January-2023.pdf

Rolfe, G., Freshwater, D. and Jasper, M. (2001) *Critical Reflection for Nursing and the Helping Professions: A User's Guide*. Basingstoke: Palgrave.

Schön, D. (1992) *The Reflective Practitioner: How Professionals Think in Action*. London: Routledge.

The Care Collective (2020) *The Care Manifesto: The Politics of Interdependence*. London: Verso Books.

University of Hull (n.d.) *Reflective Writing: Reflective Frameworks*. https://libguides.hull.ac.uk/reflectivewriting/reflection3

CHAPTER 16

Research and Evaluation

Richard Coaten and Maria Pasiecznik Parsons

Introduction

This chapter defines and outlines the purpose of research and evaluation and how it is carried out in order to highlight different approaches and methods and their relative strengths and limitations in conducting research in arts for health, particularly creative arts for dementia. This is a large subject that includes different philosophical ideas about the nature of knowledge, how the social world is viewed, what ought to be studied and in what way. Our summary risks caricaturing the differences between quantitative and qualitative research, but we endeavour to explain key ideas and terms and provide examples of research studies and ample references. We encourage Creative Health Practitioners (CHPs), whether they are less familiar with research and evaluation or more experienced, to use the learning points about how to upskill and the supplementary resources to inform and improve their practice.

As this handbook shows, there is now a wealth of research and evaluation studies that both show the tangible benefits of engagement in creative arts for people living with dementia and guide and shape practice and policy. However, given the complexity of arts-based interventions, coupled with limited resources, many studies are small and take place within short time frames, hence the difficulty of confirming (or proving) that the arts 'work'. As noted in Chapter 1, demands for evidence have increased, particularly because 'robust evidence becomes central to any effort to translate promising demonstration projects into sustained programmes of work through commissioning by the public sector' (Clift 2012 p.123), hence the impetus to use methods that provide better quality evidence of effect and impact in creative health.

Research and evaluation are distinct yet complementary methods of inquiry that have different purposes and methods. In this context, they are used to better understand the complexities involved in creative health interventions with people living with dementia. In a nutshell, *research* aims to generate new knowledge and contribute to academic discourse and *prove* something, while *evaluation* is more focused on assessing the effectiveness of an intervention or, more often, a specific programme, i.e. to *improve* something. The results or outputs of both research and evaluation are used to help develop the evidence base for, in this instance, creative arts, leading to more effective interventions, programmes and services. Quantitative and qualitative research approaches and methods are used in both research and evaluation, but increasingly, mixed methods are favoured in 'striking a balance between scientific rigour and the flexibility and creativity essential to arts' and (really) capturing the benefits of the arts (Fancourt 2017 p.198).

Context

The exponential growth of using creative arts as a medium for maintaining and improving the health and wellbeing of people living with dementia is due, in no small part, to the demand for evidence of its effectiveness (Schneider 2018, 2023). This has contributed to the steady increase in the number of research studies in arts for dementia, especially since 2010 (Manji and Fallavollita 2022), that have stimulated interest in the field and development of projects and programmes. Contemporary research continues a biomedical focus on reduction of behavioural symptoms, for example, apathy, cognition, depression and mood (Beard 2012) in ways that emulate evidence-based medical research (Manji and Fallavollita 2022). Schneider agrees:

> Dementia research has largely regarded the arts through an "instrumental" lens. They are treated as complex, psychosocial interventions, akin to a pharmacological or psychological treatment. Experimental science has a clear pipeline for the development, testing and implementation of such interventions, which research into the arts in dementia has mostly followed. (Schneider 2023 p.1861)

Taking a broader view, Vernooij-Dassen *et al.* (2019) call for an integrated biomedical and psychosocial approach in research, whilst Fancourt (2017 p.103) proposes using a 'problem solving solution model' that enables researchers to make choices about relevant methods.

Research approaches and methods

Research in the field of arts and dementia involves a structured and systematic process of inquiry that aims to generate new knowledge, theories or insights about a particular aspect of practice and/or policy. Simply put, the process involves deciding on a focus or problem, developing the research question(s) related to it and choosing a strategy or methodology that helps answer the questions. A review of the literature is essential to be able to situate the research in a body of knowledge where shortcomings or a gap has been found. Following this, a specific approach to the conduct of the research and tools (methodology) are identified to answer the question(s)/measure change. It also involves arranging the practical elements, collecting the data, preparing and carrying out analysis and reporting what has been discovered (disseminated) and its relevance to the field (Robson 1993).

Crucially, and this cannot be overstated, people with lived experience of the condition and their carers should be fully involved in research and evaluation. 'Hearing' the voices of people living with dementia has become a core consideration in developing research, policy and care practice both in the UK and worldwide. Yet until relatively recently, these 'voices' were overlooked or ignored in care practice (Killick and Benson 1994), service development (Goldsmith 1996) and research (Wilkinson 2001). Participants living with the condition were often pathologized, and difficulties were perceived in involving them.

Nevertheless, there are ethical requirements for safeguarding research participants that need to be adhered to, beginning with the need for participants to give their consent to participate, a decision that may be harder to make if the person has a cognitive impairment. The Health Research Authority is tasked in England with protecting and promoting the interests of patients and the public in health and social care research, doing this in combination with independent Research Ethics Committees (RECs) (Health Research Authority 2025).

NHS RECs review applications in England in order to protect the rights, safety, dignity and wellbeing of research participants. The Four Nations Policy Leads Group provides a coordinated research approvals system and consistent policy and good practice standards for health and social care research in the UK. Some researchers, however, report that proposed studies involving people living with dementia are often intensely scrutinised and that research ethics processes are lengthy and 'paternalistic', as people living with the condition are perceived to be particularly 'vulnerable' and in need of 'protecting' (Soofi 2022). However, Ludwin and Capstick (2017) found that residents in a care home where they were carrying out an ethnographic study had a higher capacity for research participation than assessed at the outset.

Nevertheless, there has been a welcome shift from research 'on' to research 'with' people living with dementia. Many national organisations and bodies have put in place systems and processes to support partnerships between researchers and the public to shape research projects and to facilitate

Patient and Public Involvement (PPI). For example, the Alzheimer's Society Research Network includes lay members – people living with dementia and carers – who are involved in reviewing grant applications to the charity.

The National Institute of Health Research (NIHR) research systems, services and processes are UK-wide, and it coordinates and supports PPI in England through Applied Research Collaborations (ARCs). Members of the public – including carers who are knowledgeable, for example, about dementia care – contribute to the review of NIHR applications. Applicants co-designing research have to provide evidence of the authentic involvement of the person living with the condition and/or family carer(s) throughout all research stages, which, crucially, helps real-world relevance and application in terms of practice through to dissemination (Bechard *et al.* 2022, Robson 1993).

At the same time, groups and organisations that advocate with and for people with lived experience have led a bottom-up approach to their inclusion and involvement in participatory research (Williams *et al.* 2020, Innes *et al.* 2021), supporting the development of experts by experience as co-researchers (Kowe 2022). Co-research benefits the quality of research and research outputs, but it requires additional resources, particularly costs and time for training for both researchers and lay researchers to ensure that the involvement of the latter is meaningful and effective throughout the process (Mockford *et al.* 2012, Miah *et al.* 2020).

Qualitative research

A key decision in research methodology is what methods to use to collect and analyse data. Studies that aim to understand aspects of the experience of people living with dementia generally use qualitative methods to study and understand the social world, to examine people's experiences, interactions, perspectives and behaviours and to generate theories/ideas to explain what is discovered. Research methods include interviews, focus groups, questionnaires and observation. Their suitability for people living with dementia depends on individual ability and level of cognitive impairment. Many factors can positively contribute to the inclusion of people living with dementia (Niner *et al.* 2023), including adaptations and modification of qualitative methods described by Conway *et al.* (2023 p.2005) as 'supportive changes, such as promoting comfort through using a familiar facilitator, to more extensive modifications, such as using photograph prompts and novel methods'.

Qualitative research methods such as ethnographic and emancipatory approaches are being widely used in 'field research' with people living with dementia in neighbourhoods and in care homes (Ludwin and Capstick 2017). Generic studies whereby family carers and their relatives act as co-researchers

(Birt *et al.* 2023) provide rich insights for CHPs into how people living with the condition maintain their personhood in social settings. Opportunities to use digital technology have empowered people living with dementia and supported their active participation in collecting and analysing data through the use of digital devices and techniques including a flipcam (Capstick 2011), photo-elicitation techniques with individuals and carers (Wang 2023) and photography (see Chapter 12 of this book). These 'creative, sensory and embodied research methods typically involve techniques that conceptually bring individuals "into" the research, thus affording an expressive capacity that traditional methods do not' (Fleetwood-Smith, Tischler and Robson 2022 p.263); however, there are resource implications in using innovative qualitative research methods, and detailed planning is required (Phillipson and Hammond 2018).

One of the strengths of using creative arts is that diverse individuals with different abilities can be involved on multiple levels by practitioners using a range of artistic disciplines channelled into various activities in a variety of settings. Unsurprisingly, therefore, what happens during a participatory arts session is complex and difficult to 'unpack' in terms of 'active ingredients', to measure and indeed to 'prove', a challenge taken up by Warran, Burton and Fancourt (2022) who co-produced research that has identified how arts engagement may activate causal mechanisms that affect health and wellbeing outcomes. The output of their research – the INgredients iN ArTs in hEalth (INNATE) Framework and toolkit – aims to support the design, implementation and evaluation of arts in health activities.

Quantitative research

Quantitative research uses the natural science model, tests theories and hypotheses and involves the collection of quantitative (mainly) numerical data that is analysed and reported in terms of statistics. It is used in many scientific research fields, particularly in clinical trials testing new drugs and in health research where evidence is graded in terms of certain quality criteria. The most reliable studies, considered to include the best evidence for making decisions about health care, are Randomised Controlled Trials (RCTs), which are regarded as the 'gold standard' (Hariton and Locascio 2018) of evidence-based research, usually conducted using comparative, controlled experiments. However, this type of research is not good at measuring relationship variables, such as the impact of a Creative Practitioner's (CP) personality on the outcomes of an arts session for its participants. Using an RCT to study the personal as relationship variable has to be in subservience to the content of the session itself. This frame establishes that the intervention itself is what makes the difference to measurable outcomes rather than the CP's or Creative Arts Therapist's (CAT) style of facilitation and/or relationship to group members.

The key to RCTs is the control group. A control is a similar group to the intervention group and involves an activity similar to what the intervention group might have done if they were not involved in the arts session. Both intervention and controls receive the same tests and measures over the same time frame, and causal relationships between the two can be identified, controlled for and analysed. Crucially, biases have to be accounted for and controlled; one way of doing this is to randomise the selection of participants to either intervention or control. Once statistical methods or analysis have been applied to the results, generalisations can be made applicable or not to the general population – the population size of the sample may be too small to be statistically useful or applicable. These rigorous studies are very expensive and may result in answers that appear equivocal or inconclusive. They also require rigorous planning, coordination and execution to minimise biases and other confounding variables (Bondemark and Ruf 2015).

Co-editor Richard's own doctoral studies employed a combination of both quantitative and qualitative methods including Narrative, Phenomenology, Ethnology, Grounded Theory and Case Study, known collectively as mixed-methods research (Coaten 2009). This research strategy can often contribute to a more complete account of the topic being researched and is increasingly used in arts and culture research, especially in response to the demand amongst commissioners and funders for evidenced-based studies.

Better evidence for creative arts in dementia

Systematic reviews are a research method that aims to gather and evaluate all empirical evidence in a specific area and use that evidence to draw conclusions that summarise the research. Reviews by Cowl and Gaugler (2014), Emblad and Mukaetova-Ladinska (2021), Manji and Fallavollita (2022), a Letrondo et al. (2023) focus on various aspects of creative arts for dementia and report several positive and promising findings. However, they highlight a range of limitations regarding the size of the studies, hence the extent to which research can be generalised to a broader population. Other limitations can influence research reliability – can we obtain and reproduce the same results under the same conditions? – and a different question about research validity: do the results really represent what they are supposed to measure? Finally, what about long-term (longitudinal) health benefits of arts-based interventions?

Fancourt et al. (2023) drew attention to the limitations of the results of a previous high-level mapping of evidence for the health benefits of the arts, including prevention, health promotion and managing and treating illness. This study by Fancourt and Finn (2019) gathered and analysed over 3000 studies from diverse disciplines produced in the last two decades. Its limitations included the size of many studies, small samples of people with the same or similar characteristics and time-limited programmes. Follow-ups, where they occurred, were often less than one year long.

In a further study, Fancourt *et al.* (2023) therefore sought to address the lack of long-term evidence in order to demonstrate health outcomes at population level, over longer periods of time, by using cohort studies. These follow representative groups of people over decades and regularly gather data from participants across the life course. Analysis enables researchers to identify factors that might influence outcomes in later life.

Several cohort studies that include responses to questions about arts and cultural involvement provided longitudinal results. Analysis of these studies enables researchers to show, for example, that 'lower social interaction was associated with an increased risk of developing dementia' (*ibid.* p.13) and that watching television is associated with adverse cognitive and physical health effects such as poorer verbal memory and more sedentary behaviours. A number of findings are qualified, given the difficulty of identifying when cognitive decline began, but researchers assert that 'arts can provide opportunities for social interaction, movement, and activity and could therefore have a role in mitigating some of the behavioural factors that are associated with increased risk of dementia' (*ibid.* p.18). This claim is supported by a global investigation of modifiable risk factors for dementia, whose findings highlight the importance of maintaining social health and cognitive reserve in various ways, including meaningful activities and social engagement (Livingston *et al.* 2024).

Research examples

Research is usually carried out through partnerships between university-based researchers and experts in the fields of ageing, arts and humanities, psychologists, doctoral students and CATs. Larger projects and programmes in creative arts are often funded by grants from funding bodies such as the Arts and Humanities Research Council (AHRC), national arts councils and the National Lottery Heritage Fund. Final reports about the outcome or product of research are a mandatory output.

The Museums on Prescription (2014–2017) project (Veall *et al.* 2017), funded by the AHRC, was carried out by researchers at University College London and Canterbury Christ Church University. The project helped connect older people at risk of social isolation (referred through health services, local authorities, adult social care and third-sector organisations) with partner museums in London and Kent via social prescription schemes. Participants took part in ten weekly two-hour museum sessions that included a variety of 20–30 minute activities (for example, talks, behind-the-scenes tours, gallery visits, object handling and discussion, collections-inspired creative activities and co-production of exhibitions and museum guides).

The research investigated the processes, practices, value and impact of social prescription schemes with specific reference to museums using a range of methods to assess the benefits of Museums on Prescription for older people. A mixed-methods approach was used to assess wellbeing and social inclusion, qualitative evaluation was used to thematically analyse weekly diaries of participants including carers and facilitators and in-depth interviews took place at the programme end, with three- and six-month follow-ups. Quantitative findings demonstrated statistically significant improvements in psychological wellbeing over the duration of programmes using the UCL Museums Wellbeing Measure. Findings included a range of benefits such as the importance of a sense of belonging and improved quality of life.

Evaluation

Evaluation is a systematic process of assessing the effectiveness of an intervention, project, programme or policy. It involves the collection and analysis of data to determine whether or not intended aims and objectives were achieved. These can include participant outcomes such as quality of life and wellbeing, as well as broader aims such as determining the influence of staff culture on care practice. Beyond judging whether whatever was carried out achieved its aim and objectives, an evaluation seeks to discover the key factors that contributed to its achievement or that were implicated in its failure to achieve desired results in order to inform decisions and/or make recommendations. Findings are typically reported to programme commissioners, who are usually the funders and stakeholders.

A range of research methods can be used, including surveys, interviews, observation, data analysis and, increasingly, methods to evaluate cost effectiveness such as Social Return on Investment (SROI) in order to calculate the social value of investment and provide value-for-money analysis and options (Social Value UK 2014). Calculating the cost effectiveness of aspects of arts for health requires specialist skills and training, and few studies have commanded sufficient resources to conduct these. The National Centre for Creative Health (NCCH) ran a roundtable on evidencing value for money and cost effectiveness in creative health projects (NCCH, 2023a). The NCCH Creative

Health Review (2023b p.92) includes a list of UK arts-for-health studies that employed SROI to measure social value. This includes a national study of arts for dementia in England and Wales that used economic evaluation as part of its mixed-methods research (Windle *et al.* 2016) but concluded that 'further rigorous economic evaluation is desirable to improve our understanding in this area' (NCCH 2023b p.94).

Creative health interventions are often complex, and it is helpful to look at some examples of high-quality evaluations. A comprehensive introduction to the process and planning of evaluation can be found in Daykin (2016), which provides a framework and guidance for developing and reporting project activities. It is very detailed, so a beginning practitioner is advised to work with an advisory group or with peer support to learn how to use the systematic approach and steps to be accomplished. The Culture, Health and Wellbeing Alliance (CHWA) offers a range of resources about research and evaluation. The Baring Foundation's ten-year arts and older people's programme (2010–2020) supported a large number of arts and culture organisations, whose project and programme evaluations are downloadable from the website, including a much-needed review of arts and creative ageing projects in underserved communities (Lowe 2020). Dare to Imagine (Wilson *et al.* 2023) offers a robust evaluation of artists in residence in Essex care homes.

An evaluation of Age Exchange: RADIQL™ model

Age Exchange's Reminiscence Arts programme focuses on using creativity to explore the personal histories of older people, including those living with dementia, in order to enrich caring relationships in the present. Age Exchange developed a support methodology called RADIQL™ (Reminiscence Arts and Dementia, Impact on Quality of Life) that aims to reduce levels of isolation, loneliness, unhappiness and depression for older people. It uses a personalised and relationship-centred reminiscence method centred on each individual's interests and life history, set within a social context, and a variety of creative art forms and memory methods to connect people to their present, social space and others around them. Along with an intensive programme of activity for participants with dementia, RADIQL includes a structured training and mentoring programme for care staff that supports them to apply Reminiscence Arts activities and principles to their practice.

Between 2012 and 2015, Age Exchange ran a three-year RADIQL programme of weekly groups and one-to-one interventions with older residents living in 12 residential care homes and continuing care units in Southwark and Lambeth, South London. The aim of the programme was to develop a high-quality, evidence-based conceptual and pedagogic framework for social care workers and art practitioners that would be delivered to people living with dementia in care homes. A programme evaluation to ascertain the impact of Reminiscence Arts on the wellbeing of people with dementia was carried out using quantitative, arts-based research methods and Dementia Care Mapping (DCM). Researchers at Royal Holloway, University of London produced a qualitative report (Nicholson *et al.* 2015) and a quantitative report (Cole, Keating and Grant 2015). Simetrica undertook a Cost Effectiveness Analysis (CEA) to produce a full assessment of the effectiveness of the RADIQL programme (Fujiwara and Lawton 2015).

Major findings were that the wellbeing of participants with dementia increased by 42% and positive behaviour increased by 25% as a result of taking part in Reminiscence Arts activity; there was also improvement in quality of life and social health, and cost effectiveness results demonstrated cost savings.

Conclusion

This chapter examined research and evaluation in the field of arts and dementia, highlighting the importance of involving people living with dementia in all stages of research and formal (PPI) mechanisms for doing so, as well as inclusive methods. It sketched out key aspects of the research process, touched on methodology, examined quantitative and qualitative methods and provided examples of research and evaluation studies. There is now stronger evidence for the health and wellbeing effects of arts and culture, including long-term effects, and a firmer base for asserting that:

> Among older adults, in addition to psychological benefits, the arts have protective associations against cognitive decline, dementia incidence, and multiple aspects of physical health and functioning including frailty, chronic pain, and disability, as well as better perceptions of ageing. Even lifespan is associated; those who are culturally engaged having a lower mortality risk. (Fancourt *et al.* 2023 p.49)

The publication of the APPG AHW report (2017) marks a sea change in relation to how creative health is perceived, and research continues to play a key part. The NCCH's leadership is crucial in joining up communities of lived experience, practice and research and making headway in responding to Lord Howarth's fundamentally important question: '...why, if there is so much evidence of the efficacy of the arts in health and social care, it is so little appreciated and acted upon' (*ibid.* p.6).

LEARNING POINTS

- Use the chapter's research and evaluation references to upskill yourself.

- Keep a journal to help you plan, run, evaluate and reflect on your work. There are various resources that can help you develop evaluation skills to plan and carry out evaluation of your work – use the resources listed below to start simply and build your confidence and resource bank.

- Record what you do in a journal, for example, write out a session plan/s, including aims and objectives and how you are going to evaluate what you do. Add a narrative of your experience, pen pictures of participants and their responses and reflect on your experience. Use the reflective cycle to do this in a systematic way. If you are going to work with a group over time, involve participants in co-designing the session and gather feedback and biographical information that can help you tailor what you do to their interests, needs and diverse and intersecting identities. Collect and record basic statistical information about participants and attendance. Journal contents may also be used to populate research and/or evaluation and be written up. Remember that whatever you do in terms of research and evaluation is a contribution to your own learning and development – as it is to the field when you are able to get your work published!

- Visit CHWA to access a range of useful resources, including on research and evaluation: www.culturehealthandwellbeing.org.uk/resources/research-and-evaluation

- How might you evaluate what you do? Try visiting: www.culturehealthandwellbeing.org.uk/i-want-evaluate-my-work

- Research is typically published as an article in an academic journal, often online, where it might be available freely via Google Scholar or PubMed, though some online academic journals have payment firewalls and only offer article abstracts. Nevertheless, abstracts are usually short, clear summaries of the article and include key recommendations or results from a research study.

- Student research produced in UK and global universities can be accessed via their research repositories: https://v2.sherpa.ac.uk/opendoar. For example, Canterbury Christ Church University staff and students upload their research to: https://repository.canterbury.ac.uk

- The Centre for Cultural Value has a comprehensive website that offers resources for research and evaluation: www.culturehive.co.uk/research-and-evaluation-practice and a free online course: www.cultural-value.org.uk/evaluation-arts-culture-heritage-online-course

- The Centre for Cultural Value evaluation course can also be accessed along with hundreds of free courses on many different aspects of research and evaluation at FutureLearn: www.futurelearn.com

- Join your local university library as a public member.

- Join Dementia Community. *The Journal of Dementia Care* always includes research and evaluation articles, often about creative arts. Events are posted on the website, including free quarterly webinars featuring researchers and an annual conference: https://journalofdementiacare.co.uk

- Research and evaluation are presented at conferences such as Dementia Community's UK Dementia Congress, British Society of Gerontology and Alzheimer's Europe.

- Check out *Dementia and Imagination* – a short guide for artists and others who plan to deliver arts-based activities with people who are living with dementia. It provides a set of useful ideas and recommendations distilled from a robust research project, setting out some foundations for developing visual arts projects with and for people affected by dementia: www.artsforhealth.org/resources/dementia-and-imagination.pdf

References

APPG AHW (All-Party Parliamentary Group on Arts, Health and Wellbeing) (2017) *Creative Health: The Arts for Health and Wellbeing.* https://ncch.org.uk/appg-ahw-inquiry-report

Beard, R. (2012) 'Art therapies and dementia care: A systematic review.' *Dementia International Journal of Social Research and Practice* 11, 633–656.

Bechard, L., McGilton, K., Middleton, L., Chertkow, H., Sivananthan, S. and Bethell J. (2022) 'Engaging people with lived experience of dementia in research perspectives from a multi-disciplinary research network.' *Canadian Geriatrics Journal* 25, 3, 254–261.

Birt, L., Charlesworth, G., Moniz-Cook, E., Leung, P. *et al.* (2023) '"The dynamic nature of being a person": An ethnographic study of people living with dementia in their communities.' *The Gerontologist* 63, 8, 1320–1329.

Bondemark, L. and Ruf, S. (2015) 'Randomized controlled trial: The gold standard or an unobtainable fallacy?' *Eortho* 37, 457–461.

Capstick, A. (2011) 'Travels with a flipcam: Bringing the community to people with dementia in a day care setting through visual technology.' *Visual Studies* 26, 2, 142–147.

Clift, S. (2012) 'Creative arts as a public health resource: Moving from practice-based research to evidence-based practice.' *Perspectives in Public Health* 132, 3, 120–127.

Coaten, R. (2009) 'Building Bridges of Understanding: The Use of Embodied Practices with Older People with Dementia and their Care Staff as Mediated by Dance Movement Psychotherapy.' Unpublished Doctoral Thesis, Research Repository, University of Roehampton. https://pure.roehampton.ac.uk/portal/en/studentTheses/building-bridges-of-understanding

Cole, L., Keating, F. and Grant, R. (2015) *Reminiscence Arts and Dementia Care: Impact on Quality of Life, 2012–2015: Quantitative Evaluation Final Report, 2015.* Royal Holloway, University of London. www.eyesociation.org/AgeExchange/RADIQL%20Quantative%20Evaluation%20Final%20Report.pdf

Conway, E., MacEachen, E., Middleton, L. and McAiney, C. (2023) 'Use of adapted or modified methods with people with dementia in research: A scoping review.' *Dementia* 22, 8, 1994–2023.

Cowl, A. and Gaugler, J. (2014) 'Efficacy of creative arts therapy in treatment of Alzheimer's Disease and dementia: A systematic literature review.' *Activities, Adaptation and Aging* 38, 4, 281–330.

Daykin, N. (2016) *Arts for Health and Wellbeing. An Evaluation Framework.* London: Public Health England. https://assets.publishing.service.gov.uk/government/uploads/system/uploads/attachment_data/file/496230/PHE_Arts_and_Health_Evaluation_FINAL.pdf

Emblad, S. Y. M. and Mukaetova-Ladinska, E. B. (2021) 'Creative art therapy as a non-pharmacological intervention for dementia: A systematic review.' *Journal of Alzheimer's Disease Reports* 5, 1, 353–364.

Fancourt, D. (2017) *Arts in Health: Designing and Researching Interventions.* Oxford: Oxford University Press.

Fancourt, D. and Finn, S. (2019) *What Is the Evidence on the Role of the Arts in Improving Health and Well-Being? A Scoping Review.* Health Evidence Network (HEN) Synthesis Report 67. Copenhagen: WHO Regional Office for Europe.

Fancourt, D., Bone, J. K., Bu, F., Mak, H. W. and Bradbury, A. (2023) *The Impact of Arts and Cultural Engagement on Population Health: Findings from Major Cohort Studies in the UK and USA 2017–2022.* London: UCL. https://sbbresearch.org/wp-content/uploads/2023/03/Arts-and-population-health-FINAL-March-2023.pdf

Fleetwood-Smith, R., Tischler, V. and Robson, D. (2022) 'Using creative, sensory and embodied research methods when working with people with dementia: A method story.' *Arts & Health* 14, 3, 263–279.

Fujiwara, D. and Lawton, R. (2015) *Evaluation of the Reminiscence Arts and Dementia: Impact on Quality of Life (RADIQL) Programme in Six Care Homes.* London: Simetrica Ltd. www.eyesociation.org/AgeExchange/RADIQL%20CEA.pdf

Goldsmith, M. (1996) *Hearing the Voice of People with Dementia.* London: Jessica Kingsley Publishers.

Hariton, E. and Locascio, J. J. (2018) 'Randomised controlled trials: The gold standard for effectiveness research.' *BJOG: An International Journal of Obstetrics and Gynaecology* 125, 13, 1716.

Health Research Authority (2025) What we do. www.hra.nhs.uk/about-us/what-we-do

Innes, A., Smith, S. K., Wyatt, M. and Bushell, S. (2021) '"It's just so important that people's voices are heard": The dementia associate panel.' *Journal of Aging Studies* 59, 100958.

Killick, J. and Benson, S. (1994) 'There's so much to hear, when you stop and listen to individual voices.' *Journal of Dementia Care* 2, 5, 16–17.

Kowe, A., Panjaitan, H., Klein, O. A., Boccardi, M. *et al.* (2022) 'The impact of participatory dementia research on researchers: A systematic review.' *Dementia: International Journal of Social Research and Practice* 21, 3, 1012–1031.

Letrondo, P. A., Ashley, S. A., Flinn, A., Burton, A., Kador, T. and Mukadam N. (2023) 'Systematic review of arts and culture-based interventions for people living with dementia and their caregivers.' *Ageing Research Reviews* 83, 101793.

Livingston, G., Huntley, J., Lui, Y., Costafreda, S. G, *et al.* (2024) 'Dementia prevention, intervention, and care: 2024 report of the Lancet standing Commission.' *The Lancet* 404, 10452, 572–628.

Lowe, H. (ed.) (2020) *On Diversity and Creative Ageing, A Selection of Projects Bringing Arts and Creativity to Underserved Older Communities.* London: The Baring Foundation. https://cdn.baringfoundation.org.uk/wp-content/uploads/BF-%C2%AD-Creative-ageing-and-diversity_WEB_LR.pdf

Ludwin, K. and Capstick, A. (2017) *Ethnography in Dementia Care Research: Observations on Ability and Capacity. SAGE Research Methods Cases: Ethnography.* London: SAGE.

Manji, I. and Fallavollita, P. (2022) 'A brief report on reviews of existing creative art-based interventions in dementia care from 2010 to 2020.' *Frontiers in Aging 3*, 865533.

Miah, J., Parsons, S., Lovell, K., Starling, B., Leroi, I. and Dawes, P. (2020) 'Impact of involving people with dementia and their care partners in research: A qualitative study.' *BMJ Open* 1–12, 10:e039321.

Mockford, C., Staniszewska, S., Griffiths, F. and Herron-Marx, S. (2012) 'The impact of patient and public involvement on UK NHS health care: A systematic review.' *International Journal for Quality in Health Care 24*, 1, 28–38.

National Centre for Creative Health (2023a) Cost-effectiveness, evidencing value for money and funding models roundtable. https://ncch.org.uk/blog/cost-effectiveness-evidencing-value-for-money-funding-models-roundtable

National Centre for Creative Health (2023b) Cost and value – the economics of creative health. https://ncch.org.uk/uploads/page/Cost-and-Value-%E2%80%93-the-Economics-of-Creative-Health.pdf

Nicholson, H., Keating, F., Cole, L., Lloyd, J. and Grant, R. (2015) *Reminiscence Arts and Dementia Care: Impact on Quality of Life, 2012–2015: A Final Report of the Evaluation.* London: Royal Holloway, University of London. www.eyesociation.org/AgeExchange/RADIQL%20RHUL%20Final%20Report.pdf

Niner, S., Bran, F., Mohan, D. and Warren, N. (2023) 'Evaluating the extent of participation of people living with dementia in research.' *International Journal of Qualitative Methods 22*. https://doi.org/10.1177/16094069231211247

Phillipson, L. and Hammond, A. (2018) 'More than talking: A scoping review of innovative approaches to qualitative research involving people with dementia.' *International Journal of Qualitative Methods 17*, 1.

Robson, C. (1993) *Real World Research: A Resource for Social Scientists and Practitioner-Researchers.* Oxford, UK and Cambridge, USA: Blackwell.

Schneider J. (2018) 'The arts as medium for care and self-care in dementia: Arguments and evidence.' *International Journal of Environmental Research and Public Health 15*, 6, 1151.

Schneider, J. (2023) 'The arts in dementia: Instrumental and experiential perspectives.' *Aging & Mental Health 27*, 10, 1861–1863.

Social Value UK (2024) *Social Return on Investment, Standards and Guidance.* https://social-valueuk.org/standards-and-guidance

Soofi. H. (2022) 'Ethical aspects of facilitating the recruitment of people with dementia for clinical trials: A call for further debate.' *British Journal of Clinical Pharmacology 88*, 1, 22–26.

Veall, D. *et al.* (2017) *Museums on Prescription: A Guide to Working with Older People.* Museums on Prescription. https://culturehealthresearch.wordpress.com/museums-on-prescription

Vernooij-Dassen, M., Moniz-Cook, E., Verhey, F., Chattat, R. *et al.* (2019) 'Bridging the divide between biomedical and psychosocial approaches in dementia research: the 2019 INTERDEM manifesto.' *Ageing & Mental Health 25*, 2, 206–212.

Wang, A. H. (2023) '"I took the photograph just to show you a little bit of perspective": Photo-elicitation interviewing with family caregivers in the dementia context.' *Forum Qualitative Sozialforschung Forum: Qualitative Social Research 24*, 1.

Warran, K., Burton, A. and Fancourt, D. (2022) 'What are the active ingredients of "arts in health" activities? Development of the INgredients iN ArTs in hEalth (INNATE) Framework.' (Version 1; peer review: 1 approved, 1 approved with reservations.) *Wellcome Open Research 7*, 10.

Wilkinson, H. (2001) *The Perspectives of People with Dementia: Research Methods and Motivations.* London: Jessica Kingsley Publishers.

Williams, V., Webb, J., Read, S., James, R. and Davis, H. (2020) 'Future lived experience: Inclusive research with people living with dementia.' *Qualitative Research 20*, 5, 721–740.

Wilson, C., Dadswell, A., Bungay, H. and Munn-Giddins, C. (2023) *Dare to Imagine: Artists and Care Home Staff Working Together to Embed Creativity in Care Homes. Artists' Residencies in Care Homes Programme 2019–23.* Magic Me and Anglia Ruskin University. https://flipbooks.gs-cdn.co.uk/aru-magic-me

Windle, G., Newman, A., Burholt, V., Woods, B. *et al.* (2016) 'Dementia and imagination: A mixed-methods protocol for arts and science research.' *BMJ Open 6*, 11, e011634.

CHAPTER 17

The Working Lives of Freelance Creative Health Practitioners

Rewards and Challenges

Maria Pasiecznik Parsons with Kaya Green, Helen Shearn, Kate Wilkinson and Richard Coaten

Introduction

This chapter examines the working lives of freelance Creative Health Practitioners (CHPs); it contributes to research and informs policy and practice initiatives that aim to address aspects of their precarious work. This comes to mind when, as the self-employed chief executive of Creative Dementia Arts Network (CDAN), I (Maria) respond to the most frequent enquiry the charity receives: 'Please can you advise me about becoming an arts practitioner working with people living with dementia – what training do I need, what's the pay like and how flexible is the work?' I always acknowledge that the work offers practitioners autonomy and flexibility but is precarious and, whilst deeply fulfilling, impacts on the emotional and psychological health of freelance CHPs whose needs for affective support are largely unmet.

Building on an examination of the creative health workforce (Chapter 14) and self-care and support in creative health practice (Chapter 15), the chapter presents insights into the working lives of freelance CHPs, including Community Practitioners (CPs) and Creative Arts Therapists (CATs). The literature review supplements a dearth of research about freelance practitioners in creative health, with studies of freelancers in the cultural and creative industries showing that, notwithstanding different occupational goals and outputs, their work-based experiences are largely congruent.

Interpretative Phenomenological Analysis (IPA) is used to examine the working lives of an art therapist, a community musician and an arts, health, heritage and wellbeing consultant, who all work or have worked with people living with dementia. An analysis of transcribed semi-structured interviews with participants identifies five superordinate themes: becoming a freelancer, managing and maintaining work, psychological and emotional impact, self-care and support, and connecting and learning. Practitioners collaborated in refining the analysis, developing conclusions and contributing to learning points.

Literature review

Whilst freelancing offers autonomy, flexibility and freedom to innovate, the work is widely acknowledged to be precarious and characterised by the 'uncertainty, instability, vulnerability and insecurity' (Hewison 2016 p.426) associated with job insecurity, low pay, long hours, limited employment rights and limited entitlement to Universal Credit and state pension (Maples *et al.* 2024). In the UK's creative and cultural industries, employers 'traditionally use part-time, project-based, freelance work to regulate jobs and manage costs' (Carey, Giles and O'Brien 2023 p.8), whilst fixed-term and/or sessional work contracts are also the standard way in which CHPs are employed by arts, health and social care organisations. These precarities, embedded within complex social, political and economic systems, reflect the structural inequalities associated with neoliberalism triggered by deregulation of labour markets (Blustein *et al.* 2024). Creative and cultural freelancers have continued to bear the brunt of employers cutting costs during successive socio-economic upheavals, including austerity, Brexit, COVID-19 (Chamberlain and Morris 2021) and the cost-of-living crisis (Maples 2024, Hancock and Tyler 2025).

There are multiple entry points into the gendered creative 'careers' workforce (Conor, Gill and Taylor 2015), with pathways contingent on age, class, sexuality, disability and ethnicity. Given that unpaid work experience and voluntary work are usually prerequisites for securing and maintaining (freelance) work (Taylor and Luckman 2021), the pathway favours individuals with social and economic resources and disadvantages many people from Black and Minority Ethnic communities and socially deprived backgrounds (NCCH 2023, Maples *et al.*, 2024). Postgraduate study in art, music, drama or dance movement psychotherapy remains a pathway to a salaried post for CATs. With more diverse backgrounds and qualifications, most CHPs pursue individualised work pathways, sometimes switching into the creative health practice later in their 30s (Gordon Nesbitt 2024). Reduced numbers of NHS posts have also contributed to more CATs becoming freelancers (Schneider 2018).

The Creative Health State of the Sector (CHP) survey (Tang 2023) provides an indicative picture of CHPs, who made up 54.5% of all respondents, of whom 72% were CPs and 18% CATs. Some 50% were self-employed, most freelancers, who worked for cultural or creative organisations, the NHS, local authorities, social care providers and Voluntary, Community and Social Enterprise (VCSE) organisations. The majority of CPs worked for small organisations, mainly charities with fewer than five permanent staff. Overall, cultural or creative organisations worked with an average of 18 freelancers per year, with 50% working with at least ten freelancers.

Freelance CHPs need to sustain a pipeline of contracts, given an average income of £9,895 per annum (*ibid.*), but like freelancers in creative and cultural industries, many often work below the national living wage, and most work for less than their standard rate and unpaid hours (*ibid.*). Pay remains low despite some 41% union membership and ample guidance about fair pay and employment practices for commissioners, employers and providers, produced by arts councils, trade unions and professional bodies (Scott, Cunningham and Sharratt 2023, Turtle Key Arts 2024).

Emotional and psychological impact

Freelancers, who often work alone, bring passion to their work; many perceive their work as a 'calling' (O'Connor 2022), which chimes with the belief of Basting (2009) in the power of arts to harness the remaining strengths of people living with dementia and bring more meaning to life through intense interpersonal engagement, co-creation and creative care. Thus, 'the making of arts can be an act of care' (Thompson 2023 p.1) as illustrated by a practice example in Chapter 2 that describes an act of profound relational care between a Dance Movement Psychotherapist (DMP) and a person living with dementia.

This example highlights the complex person-centred practice skills and knowledge that CHPs require: to be fully attuned to the person yet flexible and able to improvise whilst providing individual cognitive and/or physical support during (mainly) group sessions (Broome *et al.* 2019, Warran, Burton and Fancourt 2022). This creative practice is emotionally draining and often distressing, and '[t]he work inspires…but it also hurts' (O'Connor 2022 p.7). Moreover, many Creative Practitioners go far beyond their roles and contracts by compassionately shouldering all aspects of community projects, including hidden care costs (Belfiore 2022). Compassion also leads community-based socially engaged practitioners to remain involved with individuals well beyond the end of contracted work (Alacovska 2020).

Over long periods of time, CHPs risk burnout, especially CPs, who are more likely to work in settings where they experience isolation and marginalisation (Collard-Stokes and Yoon Irons 2022), which affects mental and often physical health (Kinman 2022), whilst the psychological consequences of emotional precarity also include stress associated with chronic uncertainty, particularly about job security, pay and income (Irvine and Rose 2022).

Self-care and support

Freelancers engaged in creative health practice need support and supervision to develop and maintain high-quality creative health practice. Despite the unremitting emotional, economic and structural precarities of arts freelancing (Padwick Jones 2012), many CHPs find it difficult to disengage from caring relationships and practice self-care (Alacovska 2020). Yet those working in contexts with older adults, including people living with dementia, have considerable unmet support needs around working with bereavement and loss, feeling fearful and threatened by participants living with dementia and processing feelings of guilt when abused by individuals affected by the condition (Fortier and Massey-Chase 2024).

CATs receive regular workplace-based clinical supervision, whilst those freelancing may be able to obtain support from their employers and make their own arrangements. Arts, health and social care employers do not generally offer supervision and support for freelance CPs, who are generally reluctant to ask for help, as they want to be seen as coping with the work (Naismith 2019, O'Connor 2022). Most are unwilling to use their own limited resources and they lose work, if they choose to meet their self-care and support needs (Tang 2023). In any case, provision is generally variable, mixed and inconsistent (Naismith 2022), resulting in many CHPs self-managing the emotional demands of working with participants living with challenging health conditions or social situations (Fortier 2023).

Acknowledging support and supervision as components of good practice, the Baring Foundation and Arts Council England (ACE) encourage organisations making funding applications to include reasonable costs for meeting staff (including freelancers) support needs (Cutler 2021, ACE 2024).

Learning and connecting

Working outside of an organisation means freelancers have to bear the risks of constructing careers and develop skills in navigating between success and failure. Most freelance CHPs find work through word of mouth, often by participating in online networks. The COVID-19 pandemic accelerated the shift from live community networks to 'network sociality', which is embedded in technology, is not bounded by location and involves social relationships that are 'informational' and focused on exchange of data and 'catching up' (Wittel 2001).

Despite Jacobs *et al.* (2019) finding no positive and direct association between career success and networking, Tang (2023) reported that the CHP survey respondents used networks to increase employability by finding resources and updating competencies, with almost 50% completing fund-raising courses and more indicating an interest in business skills training.

Research method

Interpretative Phenomenological Analysis (IPA) was used to design and conduct a study of the working lives of freelance CHPs. IPA is a qualitative research method that is idiographic, i.e. it provides researchers with a way of 'letting things speak for themselves by examining individual perspectives of study participants in their unique contexts, to examine how people make sense of their major life experiences' (Smith 1996 p.27).

A sample was secured via informal contact with freelancers known to CDAN, and three experienced participants were selected on the basis of their employment in the statutory, VCSE and/or commercial health and social care sector and work with people living with dementia. Crucially, they consented to openly sharing and reflecting on their working lives as research partici-pants and collaborators.

Kate is an experienced freelance community musician, whose mixed portfolio includes work: with people living with dementia in day centres, care homes and hospitals; with a music charity providing music sessions for learning disabled people with complex support needs; and as an animateur for a professional orchestra's community outreach programme, which includes working in community hospitals and secure mental health units.

Kaya practices as an art therapist and has worked with children and adults in various settings over 15 years. Her current portfolio combines salaried work as a lead art therapist – running a weekly art therapy group with people living with dementia for a community garden, where she is safeguarding lead – with freelance work with children at a primary school, as well as delivering clinical supervision for therapists and frontline workers.

Helen is a freelance consultant in arts, health, heritage and wellbeing. After several years as an art teacher, she retrained as an occupational therapist using the arts and then became an arts manager and strategic head of arts in mental health at an NHS trust. She developed a pioneering arts programme with wards for older patients, in partnership with South London art galleries and museums. After the post was cut, she set up her consultancy, which has included designing, facilitating and evaluating museum projects with and for people living with dementia.

Each participant received information about the research study and IPA plus a questionnaire to complete in preparation for a two-hour individual semi-structured online interview with the researcher. This aimed to understand the social lens of participants' perspectives and perceptions of their work and their choices, behaviours and experiences (Wright 2022).

Interviews were transcribed verbatim and analysed using IPA, and five superordinate themes were identified: becoming a freelancer, managing and maintaining work, psychological and emotional impact, self-care and support, and connecting and learning.

Results and discussion
Becoming a freelancer

Kate, Kaya and Helen's reflections offer a view of their motivation for beginning a career in creative health practice and the commitment and determination involved in pursuing diverse circuitous pathways, shaped by individual needs and circumstances.

Kate – driven by passion

A combination of experiencing the many positive impacts of music on the lives of people living with dementia through volunteering and a lifelong passion for music led Kate to becoming a community music practitioner. She found using music to relate to people living with dementia particularly fulfilling.

Kate and Kaya – service to others

Both drew attention to a powerful and purposeful sense of service to others. This is echoed by O'Connor (2022), who describes how study participants working in health, care and participatory settings refer to their artistic and therapeutic work with vulnerable people as 'a calling' (p.7), 'precious' (p.8), 'a privilege' (p.7) and 'a blessing' (p.7).

Helen – community capacity building

Although no longer directly practising arts with older people living with mental health needs/dementia, Helen is deeply committed to enabling communities and project partners to build community capacity through arts, health, heritage and nature, using a range of skills and consultancy roles as 'an awareness raiser', 'silo breaker', 'catalyst' and 'pollinator' to effect change.

Managing and maintaining work

Freelancers have to develop a wide range of administrative and technical skills to create and manage their work, but despite running an 'enterprise', Kaya had not completed any business skills training. Kate had completed a GCSE and further business courses, whilst Helen drew on arts management skills to assist her boundary spanning between policy and practice, health and social care and across a range of arts-related areas including heritage and nature.

Kaya encourages art therapists to be more proactive…

Kaya had combined her therapeutic and 'enterprising self' to establish an art therapy group for people living with dementia in a community garden in a city park, demonstrating her resourcefulness in joining as a volunteer, forming relationships with the staff team, introducing her idea of the group, creating a role, helping to raise funds for art therapy staff and providing student placements. She used her experience to encourage students 'to create their own opportunities and as art therapists to be proactive, rather than sending off an application form'. The British Association of Art Therapists (BAAT) Workforce Survey 2018 (Carr and McDonald 2019) largely confirms Kaya's observations that more art therapy graduates are choosing self-employment over traditional NHS work, with most assembling a part employment, part self-employment portfolio.

Psychological and emotional impact

Once they actively *become* freelancers, CHPs have to manage the psychological and emotional challenges of the work and 'the difficulty of how to balance this depth of care and connection with the self-protection that enables artists to stay well' (O'Connor 2022 p.9). Whilst Kaya and Kate attest to finding joy in working with people living with dementia, they are aware of the 'psychological intensity of the work and its proximity to death and suffering' (O'Connor 2022 p.10).

Coping with death

Kate pointed out that when practitioners arrive at a healthcare or social care setting, even one they know well, they don't know what awaits them. From time to time, staff will share the sad news that a person she has worked and developed a relationship with over a long period has died, and 'you can't fully process this in the moment as you have to continue to deliver your music session, so you need to find a way of coming to terms with the news after the session has finished.' The vulnerability of people living with dementia increases the possibility 'that you may face potentially upsetting and challenging scenarios regularly, and practitioners in this field will need to develop coping mechanisms for this'. This can be a real challenge for both practition-ers and members of the group they are facilitating.

Commitment to authentic expression

In all of her sessions, Kaya pays 'very specific attention to [participants'] authentic expression of themselves...an intense process that I am engaged and committed to as a therapist'. She feels that group members living with dementia are aware at some level that losses are inevitable. Individuals become more disabled, and they may be admitted to care homes or death may occur, but she acknowledges that '[i]t's a minor miracle them coming through the door...honestly sometimes I am lost for words that people have made it in...a testament to human strength and resilience'.

Managing and mitigating the stress of wondering where future income is coming from

The pattern of Helen's work calls for constant vigilance in terms of a work pipeline. She describes how nerve-wracking it is as a freelancer when 'you are wondering about income; so there is that kind of precariousness as some organisations take ages to decide what they are going to do'. Helen also observed that 'everything you do you have to do as there's no such thing as a back office', and like Kate, is conscious of stress around delayed payment of invoices.

Self-care and support

All participants acknowledged their self-care and support needs and met these in different ways. An experienced art therapist, Kaya is a clinical supervisor for staff and students, and she had organised a comprehensive programme of supervision and support for herself. She spoke of the impor-tance of 'demarcating personal and professional life and switching off and protecting weekends'. This was, she admitted, difficult; she had had to 'keep practising and practising' and try 'different strategies', including 'being in the moment' (which also took practice). Kaya's observation that 'everyone is going to have something that suits them' chimes with the work of Naismith (2022), who devised a support menu for practitioners, who can choose a mode that meets their needs in a way that suits their work pattern.

Kate's experience and her highly organised approach to scheduling work is not simply an efficient use of time but it also enables her to maintain her wellbeing. Ensuring much of her work is co-located (to reduce the burden of travel), her personalised support arrangements include peer support, affec-tive support and work debriefings with managers, besides playing music, singing in choirs and walking in nature.

Helen draws on her experience of support and supervision – as a supervisee, a supervisor and team leader – in developing a support programme that includes peer support with an artist with whom she has worked on topics such as boundary setting, teamwork and contracting.

Connecting and learning

In the absence of a specialist degree in creative arts and dementia, and limited continuing professional development (CPD), practitioners usually develop relevant skills and knowledge by experience (see Chapter 14). Kaya completed a post-qualifying practice learning course in creative arts and dementia abroad and developed her experience through running a community-based art group. CPD is a mandatory requirement for arts therapists, although Kaya admitted this was sometimes 'last on the list' given her focus on therapy participants and the expense of some CPD courses.

For most CHPs, CPD usually involves replacing potential paid work with training or events and forgoing income or time that might have been devoted to finding work. Kate believes investment is necessary to maintain high-quality practice and has continued to self-fund attendance at conferences, webinars, workshops and courses, such as Creative and Credible Evaluation training and facilitator training including Singing for Lung Health with The Musical Breath and Sing to Beat Parkinson's.

Helen strongly emphasised the need for consultants to stay abreast of policy and practice in arts and health by receiving online updates from relevant organisations such as the Culture, Health and Wellbeing Alliance (CHWA) London Arts and Health, and the National Centre for Creative Health (NCCH).

Freelancers are 'cut off' from the organisation/workplace that provides employees with formal and informal opportunities to meet needs relating to autonomy, competence, relatedness and connectedness, a critical social resource, especially for wellbeing (Jacobs *et al.* 2019). Kate and Kaya's local networks support their work, whilst Helen benefits from being active in national arts, culture, health and heritage networks and participating in online and in-person events that offer learning, support and contact with potential work contacts.

Discussion

I am indebted to the three study collaborators, who openly shared aspects of their working lives with me. Whilst the research involved a very small cohort of freelancers, data analysis shows that results are consistent with the literature in respect of the rewards, challenges and risks associated with freelancing, and together, these offer answers to the most frequent practitioner enquiry received by CDAN.

So why and how do these freelancers continue to work in the face of economic and emotional precarities?

Kaya is in awe of the 'human strength and resilience' of her group members with varying levels of cognitive impairment, who turn up every week and engage in art. Kate regularly experiences the joy that music can bring to hospital patients and care home residents and witnesses the positive impact on patients living with dementia, as well as their relatives and carers. Helen's therapeutic arts practice, management and multi-agency partnership experience enable her to successfully facilitate relationships and joint work involving colleagues and communities.

All use skills and knowledge to improve health and wellbeing whilst managing a huge and varied portfolio of work but are aware that 'this work hurts' (O'Connor 2022), that self-care, support and supervision are important and that the learning process is continual; for Helen, networks are the core of her work. Despite differing backgrounds and training, what emerges from the descriptions of practice is the potential for cross-collaboration between CATs and CPs (see Chapter 18).

Conclusion

The chapter has examined the working lives of freelancers, raised their profile and, overall, substantiated the research literature about the precarity of the work. Job insecurity and working conditions are unlikely to improve given ongoing economic crises. Study participants emphasised the rewards of freelance creative health practice and consultancy, highlighting autonomy and flexibility, the opportunity to use their passion and deep interest in an art form to help vulnerable individuals and communities, and the satisfaction gained from relational work.

However, they bore all the risks of self-employment themselves, including the emotional, economic and structural precarities of their working lives, beginning with finding and managing individualised and self-directed pathways, including graduate study, training and jobs that provided a springboard into their chosen occupation and role. Substantial experience and contacts enable work to be found through 'word of mouth', usually via networks, although time is also often spent 'pitching', along with juggling commissioned work and completing administration, including invoicing and getting paid.

Working with people living with dementia is often emotionally and psychologically intense. Whilst one study participant (an art therapist) benefitted from employer support for her clinical supervision, the others were responsible for securing and financing their own support. Further training and CPD were largely self-funded, and skills were developed 'on the job' in arts, health or social care settings. Online networks were key conduits for exchanging information, making contacts for work and updating knowledge and skills, particularly in creative health consultancy.

Whilst ACE has 'a pivotal role in shaping freelancers' current circumstances and future work potential [and] a potential role in more effective fund allocation' (Maples *et al.* 2024 p.70), there is an urgent need for a collective and coordinated approach to developing more work/posts in creative health, addressing the pay and conditions of freelance CHPs and meeting workforce development and practitioner support needs. This requires collaboration between sector- and service-level intermediary institutions and stakeholders at different levels and in different spheres, particularly arts councils, CHWA, NCCH and arts, culture, health and social care employers and commissioners.

LEARNING POINTS

For practitioners:

- Consider how best to maintain and develop physical, emotional, psychological and spiritual resources in order to support the resilience needed to better manage the challenges and opportunities presented in this work with vulnerable adults.
- Create support networks for yourself.
- Access supervision/reflexive practice opportunities.
- Restore resilience to cope with the precarities and challenges.
- Express, capture and publish all the learning in written form (journal)/visual methods, including social media platforms and networks.

For organisations/funding bodies/charities and foundations:

- Consider the real need to support practitioner resilience in the long term by encouraging applications that involve reflexive practice/supervision opportunities in work with vulnerable adults and other practices/creative ways to support artist/therapist resilience.

For professional arts therapy associations (art: British Association of Art Therapists (BAAT); music: British Association for Music Therapy (BAMT); drama: British Association of Dramatherapists (BADth); dance movement psychotherapy: Association for Dance and Movement Psychotherapy (ADMP) (UK):

- Consider the ways in which further collaboration and dialogue between association members and creative health colleagues may help break down the silos that exist between the two worlds (see Chapter 18), improve practice in the field generally, support resilience and increase interest that may in time both raise awareness of and increase membership in these associations.

Resources
Market research and scoping your locality

- Conduct a Strengths, Weaknesses, Opportunities Threats (SWOT) analysis to help you map and scope your local market.
- Local Joint Strategic Needs Assessments provide statistics about local populations and services for people living with dementia and carers and services commissioned.

Support for freelancers

- National arts councils. [PQ]
- National arts and health organisations in all four nations offer advice and support information online and host networks and events. These include:
    - England: Culture, Health and Wellbeing Alliance (CHWA) London Arts and Health[PQ]
    - Wales: Arts and Health and Wellbeing Network (WAHWN)
    - Scotland: Arts Culture Health and Wellbeing Scotland (ACHWS)
    - Northern Ireland: Arts, Health and Wellbeing in Northern Ireland.
- [PQ]www.artscouncil.org.uk/developing-creativity-and-culture/supporting-individual-creative-and-cultural-practitioners/resources-individuals
- https://takeart.org/artist-support
- www.a-n.co.uk/news
- https://precaritypilot.net
- www.freelancing.support/communities

Self-care and support

- Practising Well Conversations series: www.youtube.com/playlist?list=PLGLYem8BDz8tAHssdIoF613rgI7lhWZfV
- Leapers – Supporting the mental health of self-employed workers: www.leapers.co/research/2024/#chapter-respondants

Creative health training and CPD

- Culture, Health and Wellbeing Alliance (CHWA) online training course: www.culturehealthandwellbeing.org.uk/culture-health-and-wellbeing-online-training-course
- National Association of Social Prescribing (NASP) social prescribing training webinars: https://socialprescribingacademy.org.uk/events

Evaluation and impact

- Centre for Cultural Value, Leeds: www.culturehive.co.uk/evaluation-learning-space
- What works for wellbeing: www.thinknpc.org/starting-to-measure-your-impact
- Visual Arts South West evaluation guide: https://vasw.org.uk/resources/navigating-your-first-evaluation-a-starting-guide-for-artists-and-producers

Pay and employment practice

- [PQ]https://vasw.org.uk/resources/do-i-need-to-be-self-employed-as-an-artist-or-artworker
- www.artscouncil.org.uk/supporting-individual-creative-and-cultural-practitioners/resources-individuals/resources-individuals-business-skills/resources-individuals-networks-and-peer-learning
- Benefits for self-employed CHPs: www.entitledto.co.uk
- Advice for CHPs who have chronic illness: www.ipse.co.uk/advice/self-employed-health-issues

Unions

- Artists' Union England rates of pay: www.artistsunionengland.org.uk/rates-of-pay
- Musicians' Union: https://musiciansunion.org.uk
- Theatre freelancers: https://freelancersmaketheatrework.com
- Freelancers in the heritage sector: https://gem.org.uk/resource/starting-freelancer-heritage-learning
- CHWA and Creative Ageing: Development & Agency (CADA) have launched initiatives to provide active support for people from under-served communities who want to develop skills in creative health and ageing work.[PQ]

References

ACE (2024) Let's create: Delivery plan 2024–2027. www.artscouncil.org.uk/lets-create/delivery-plan-2024-2027

Alacovska, A. (2020) 'From passion to compassion: A caring inquiry into creative work as socially engaged art.' *Sociology* 54, 4, 727–744.

Basting, A. (2009) *Forget Memory: Creating Better Lives for People with Dementia*. Baltimore, MD: John Hopkins University Press.

Belfiore, E. (2022) 'Who cares? At what price? The hidden costs of socially engaged arts labour and the moral failure of cultural policy.' *European Journal of Cultural Studies* 25, 1, 61–78.

Blustein, D. L., Grzanka, P. R., Gordon, M., Smith, C. M. and Allan, B. A. (2024) 'The psychology of precarity: A critical framework.' *American Psychologist*. Advance online publication. https://doi.org/10.1037/amp0001361

Broome, E., Dening, T. and Schneider, J. (2019) 'Facilitating Imagine Arts in residential care homes: The artists' perspectives.' *Arts Health* 11, 1, 54–66.

Carey, H., Giles, L. and O'Brien, D. (2023) *The Good Work Review: Job Quality in the Creative Industries*. Newcastle: Creative Industries Policy and Evidence Centre.

Carr, S. and McDonald, A. (2019) 'The state-of-the-art: Building a positive future for art therapy through systematic research.' *International Journal of Art Therapy* 24, 2, 53–55.

Chamberlain, P. and Morris, D. (2021) *The Economic Impact of Covid-19 on the Culture, Arts and Heritage (CAH) Sector in South Yorkshire and Comparator Regions*. Sheffield: The University of Sheffield. https://cweconomics.co.uk/wp-content/uploads/2024/09/SY_CAH_Covid-19_2021.pdf

Collard-Stokes, G. and Yoon Irons, J. (2022) 'Artist wellbeing: Exploring the experiences of dance artists delivering community health and wellbeing initiatives.' *Research in Dance Education* 23, 1, 60–74.

Conor, B., Gill, R. and Taylor, S. (2015) 'Gender and creative labour.' *The Sociological Review* 63, S1, 1–22.

Cutler, D. (2021) Creatively minded and practising well. https://baringfoundation.org.uk/blog-post/creatively-minded-and-practising-well

Fortier, J. P. (2023) 'Navigating Ambiguity and Boundaries: The Experiences of Arts, Health and Wellbeing Facilitators Working with Individuals with Challenging Conditions or Situations.' Doctoral thesis. London: London School of Hygiene and Tropical Medicine.

Fortier, J. and Massey-Chase, K. (2024) *Keeping Safe: A Review of Psychosocial and Wellbeing Support Options for Creative Practitioners Working with Challenging Conditions and Circumstances*. Manchester: Arts Council England. www.artscouncil.org.uk/developing-creativity-and-culture/health-and-wellbeing/keeping-safe-report

Gordon Nesbitt, R. (2024) *Understanding Creative Health in London: The Scale, Character and Maturity of the Sector*. London: Greater London Authority and London Arts for Health. https://londonartsandhealth.org.uk/story/understanding-creative-health-in-london-the-scale-character-and-maturity-of-the-sector

Hancock P. and Tyler, M. (2025) *Performing Artists and Precarity Work in the Contemporary Entertainment Industries*. Palgrave Macmillan Open Access (eBook). https://doi.org/10.1007/978-3-031-66119-8

Hewison, K. (2016) 'Precarious Work.' In S. Edgell, H. Gottfried and E. Gartner (eds) *The SAGE Handbook of Sociology of Work and Employment*. London: SAGE.

Irvine, A. and Rose, N. (2022) 'How does precarious employment affect mental health? A scoping review and thematic synthesis of qualitative evidence from western economies.' *Work, Employment and Society* 38, 1–24.

Jacobs, S., De Vos, A., Stuer, D. and Van der Heijden, B. (2019) '"Knowing me, knowing you": The importance of networking for freelancers' careers: Examining the mediating role of need for relatedness fulfillment and employability-enhancing competencies.' *Frontiers in Psychology* 10, 2055, 1–14.

Kinman, G. (2022) *Supporting Practitioner Wellbeing*. Totnes: Dartington Trust. www.researchinpractice.org.uk/media/jf1ddhdw/supporting_practitioner_wellbeing_pg_web.pdf

Maples, H., Tyler, M., Hancock, P., Klich, R. and Unger, C. (2024) *Cultural Freelancers Study*. Colchester: University of Essex, for Arts Council England (ACE). www.artscouncil.org.uk/developing-creativity-and-culture/supporting-individual-creative-and-cultural-practitioners/creative-and-cultural-freelancers-study

Naismith, N. (2019) *Artists Practising Well*. Aberdeen: Robert Gordon University.

Naismith, N. (2022) Artists practising well conversations and support menu. www.nicolanaismith.co.uk/research-writing/practising-well-conversations-support-menu

National Centre for Creative Health (2023) Roundtable on Anti-Racism and Ethnic Diversity in Creative Health: Addressing Inequality in the Social Movement. https://ncch.org.uk/blog/anti-racism-and-ethnic-diversity-in-creative-health

O'Connor, A. (2022) 'The work hurts.' *Journal of Applied Arts & Health* 13, 1, 153–166.

Padwick Jones (2022) Artists' precarity not just about pay. https://padwickjonesarts.co.uk/artists-precarity-is-not-just-about-pay

Schneider, J. (2018) 'Music therapy and dementia care practice in the United Kingdom: A British Association for Music Therapy membership survey.' *British Journal of Music Therapy* 32, 2, 58–69.

Scott J., Cunningham, M. and Sharratt, C. (2023) *The Illustrated Fair Work*. Edinburgh: Creative Scotland. www.creativescotland.com/resources-publications/guides-toolkits/the-illustrated-fair-work-employers-guide

Smith, J. A. (1996) 'Beyond the divide between cognition and discourse: Using interpretative phenomenological analysis in health psychology.' *Psychology & Health* 11, 2, 261–271.

Tang, J. (2023) *Creative Health: UK State of the Sector Survey*. Barnsley: Culture, Health and Wellbeing Alliance. www.culturehealthandwellbeing.org.uk/uk-creative-health-sector-survey-2023

Taylor, S. and Luckman, S. (eds) (2021) *Pathways into Creative Lives*. Cham: Palgrave Macmillan.

Thompson, J. (2023) *Care Aesthetics for Artful Care and Careful Art*. Abingdon: Routledge.

Turtle Key Arts (2024) Turtle Key Arts freelancers manifesto. www.turtlekeyarts.org.uk/freelancermanifesto

Warran, K., Burton, A. and Fancourt, D. (2022) 'What are the active ingredients of "arts in health" activities? Development of the INgredients iN ArTs in hEalth (INNATE) framework.' *Wellcome Open Research* 7, 10.

Wittel, A. (2001) 'Toward a network sociality.' *Theory, Culture & Society* 18, 6, 51–76.

Wright, J. (2022) *Research Digest: The Role of the Artist in Society*. Leeds: Centre for Cultural Value. www.culturehive.co.uk/wp-content/uploads/2023/10/Research-Digest-The-Role-of-the-Artist-in-Society.pdf

A Positive Provocation – and Call for More Creative Dialogue and Collaboration Between Creative Arts in Health and Creative Arts Therapies

Richard Coaten with Maria Pasiecznik Parsons

This chapter makes a case for more creative dialogue and collaboration between creative arts in health and creative arts therapies in order to improve health and wellbeing outcomes for people living with dementia and their family carers.

The support needs of older frail people and people living with disabilities will continue to outpace capacity in health and social care resources. The contribution of the creative arts to the health and wellbeing of vulnerable groups, highlighted during the COVID-19 pandemic, is more important than ever, and we welcome increasing recognition of the value of arts in health and new policies geared to their adoption (Well-Being of Future Generations (Wales) Act 2015, NHS 2019, NHS England 2020, Dow *et al.* 2023, NCCH and APPG AHW 2023).

Pooling (scarce, relative to need) resources associated with arts in health and creative arts therapies through creative dialogue and collaboration will enable the arts to play a larger role in more integrated health and social care provision. Since such change involves all stakeholders, we examine driving and restraining factors that help and hinder creative dialogue and collaboration between practitioners at micro (practice) level, where Creative Practitioners (CPs) and Creative Arts Therapists (CATs) are located. Since such change involves all stakeholders, we examine driving and restraining factors that help and hinder creative dialogue and collaboration at three levels. For example, between practitioners at the micro (practice) level, where Creative Practitioners (CPs) and Creative Arts Therapists (CATs) are located; at the meso level, where arts, health and social care organisations are found; and, crucially, at the macro level, where NHS, infrastructure organisations, professional bodies, academic institutions, funding councils and other stakeholders operate and hold power.

In combining this assessment with insights from practice experience and drawing on national and international literature, it is clear that creative dialogue and collaboration is taking place and that creative arts are now playing a larger role in policy, driving the NHS towards '...a more integrated and person-centred approach to health and social care', as reported by the National Centre for Creative Health (NOAH 2017, 2018, NHS 2019, NHS England 2020, Cutler 2021, Sandford and Gilluley 2021, NCCH and APPG AHW 2023 p.14, Percy-Smith *et al.* 2024). So we offer the next steps, consider the implications and challenges for all stakeholders and conclude by asking all involved to be bold and seize opportunities for systems change offered in a new era of health and social care integration in order to deliver better outcomes for individuals, families and communities.

Provocation: key drivers

More creative dialogue and collaboration at all levels of arts in health will enhance the capacity and effectiveness of therapeutic and community-orientated arts in health resources at a time of increasing need. Ongoing austerity and fiscal pressures on statutory and voluntary services are also driving support for harnessing and mobilising the arts as key community assets in place-based partnerships for meeting the needs of an ageing population living longer with multiple health conditions.

The COVID-19 pandemic and lockdowns impacted on the health and wellbeing of many people living with long-term chronic illness and age-related conditions such as dementia. Face-to-face arts in health practice and programmes were suspended, with dire consequences for many practitioners and small and medium sized enterprise (SME) arts organisations. However, the crisis also highlighted how the arts met the health and emotional wellbeing needs of the population at home (Chapple *et al.* 2023), adapting delivery to public spaces and in nature (Heddon *et al.* 2021) and supporting informal carers (Armstrong *et al.* 2022) and healthcare staff (Wiltshire and Prescott 2023). The use of digital technology facilitated new partnerships between practitioners and arts, health and social care staff (Bradbury *et al.* 2021).

Policy

In the UK, the expansion of arts for social prescribing demonstrates NHS recognition of the value of the arts in meeting psychosocial and place-based needs associated with health inequalities, mental illness, loneliness and social isolation (Dow *et al.* 2023). Collaborative work at macro- and local-level systems of integrated care and treatment is being led by the NCCH, whose Creative Associates are working with Integrated Care Boards (ICBs) and supporting the development of Creative Health Hubs (Percy-Smith *et al.* 2024). This work is soon to be boosted by Creative Health Boards, a national Arts and Humanities Research Council-funded development programme led by Sheffield Hallam University (2024). In Wales, arts and health have a key role in the implementation of the Well-Being of Future Generations Act (2015), particularly around prevention. These policy shifts are facilitating more opportunities to develop new working relationships and partnerships that enhance and complement health and social care resources and services for people in need (Betts and Huet 2023).

Creative arts practice

CATs and CPs make up a diverse community of arts in health practice, as described in Chapter 1, whilst Chapters 4 and 6 illustrate the work of musicians and a poet who are CPs and Chapters 1 and 17 offer insights into the approach and practice of CATs who use movement, dance and art. Have those examples in mind as we go on to summarise the similarities and differences between them, the reasons for cleavages between the groups and how to promote more creative dialogue and collaboration.

Similarities and differences

CATs and CPs make relationships with people in need to facilitate opportunities for self-expression, enjoyment, confidence-building and meaning-making, both working one to one and in groups. The goals, content and format of these vary depending on their role, training and experience. CATs reflect on their practice with a supervisor or experienced peers; CPs working in larger organisations may well receive supervision but many freelancers do not, though some access practice support in other ways.

The groups generally work in different settings and in different cultures that reinforce differences in status, identity and power. CATs are almost all Allied Health Professionals, members of multidisciplinary teams, whose accreditation is recognised by the NHS and other commissioners, unlike CPs, who generally get paid less and whose job security and conditions of service are less secure than CATs.

A major obstacle to informal as well as formal dialogue between CPs and CATs is that, overall, they are insulated from one another and work in 'professional silos' (Betts and Huet 2023) that reduce opportunities for creative dialogue, collaboration and reciprocal learning about the nature of the work. Moss (2008) cites Daykin, who observes that '[t]here is in general a lack of understanding between creative arts therapists and arts in health practitioners about the unique contribution that each makes to improving and enhancing health services, and what they can learn from one another's practice' (p.86).

Richard, a Dance Movement Psychotherapist (DMP) (one of this chapter's authors), has communicated over the years with Professor Hilary Moss, a music therapist. Both have much experience of working as CATs in clinical settings and CPs in arts in health settings and acknowledge that their CAT training and experience was invaluable for their CP work.

Certainly, the expansion of arts in health since 2008 has to an extent addressed this lack of understanding, and some of the barriers between CATs and CPs are being dismantled with more focus on 'what [they) bring to each other' (Hume 2023 p.41) in terms of mutual support and learning. There is increasing creative dialogue and collaboration at the micro and meso level between CATs and CPs, including supervision, mentoring and reflective practice being offered for both by, for example, the Orange Collective and Flourishing Lives, Artlink's Music on the Wards and other hospital-based arts programmes that employ both CPs and CATs. Kazzum Arts employ both CATs and experienced CPs to provide arts and cultural events and training, and facilitate peer-to-peer support. CATs are collaborating with carer support groups, currently in early-stage development in North Yorkshire, to offer movement, dance and embodied practices, providing emotional support to family carers and ideas for development of coping and other strategies. If this pilot is successful, the model could be replicated elsewhere.

Macro-level collaboration

There are growing connections between arts organisations, health and social care commissioning and ICBs and macro-level organisations, including the NHS, arts in health infrastructure organisations, arts therapy professional bodies, academic institutions, funding councils and voluntary and commercial sector organisations. These stakeholders differ in their roles, functions and funding bases and in their relative power to promote (and resist) change.

Overall, the NHS integration agenda is driving collaboration and partnerships in the NHS and in local authorities around the commissioning, management and delivery of health and social care services and shifting more provision to primary and community care. This has implications for CATs (NHS England 2020) and for their professional bodies, such as the Health and Care Professions Council (HCPC), an independent body that has considerable power given that it registers CATs, regulates the profession, sets standards and quality assures their education, together with CAT professional bodies. Significantly, NHS England has recognised and is currently overseeing more collaboration between art, music and drama therapists, including allied health and psychological professions leadership, demonstrating multidisciplinary approaches to collaboration (NHS England 2020).

At the same time, increasing numbers of universities are accrediting arts in health undergraduate and postgraduate degree courses. Their graduates, who are not registered professionals, are nevertheless joining the arts and health workforce.

In the UK, the establishment of two key infrastructure organisations: the Culture, Health and Wellbeing Alliance (CHWA) funded by Arts Council England (ACE) and the NCCH, a national charity, provide the arts in health movement with strong, knowledgeable and visible leadership that is helping action Betts and Huet's (2023) call:

> ...to encourage not only a 'grass roots' approach to partnership work but also an active partnership building between arts therapies professional bodies, arts in health organizations, politicians, service providers (including the NHS), and people with experience of emotional and physical distress who have benefitted from the arts to develop a shared strategy. (p.12)

There is value in representatives of arts in health organisations, university course leaders, UK-based arts councils and arts therapy professional bodies coming together as, for example, Strategic Members of the CHWA to share their work and discuss key issues in the sector. More meetings would progress intra-sector collaboration.

Progressing more creative dialogue and collaboration

This call draws on the work of Moss (2016 p.12), who introduced 'A New Paradigm', the idea of a continuum, a concept that has made it possible to view all arts in health and social care related activity as part of an interdisciplinary continuum, from health humanities to community arts, to arts education, residencies, performances and exhibitions, through to arts in health practice and to the arts therapies. Moss (2008, 2016) also made one of the first compelling cases for creative dialogue between CPs and CATs, who, by becoming more knowledgeable about their respective practice and the ways in which they work, can bring significant results in improving mental healthcare for adults.

However, for examples of effecting macro-level change in arts and health more recently, much can be learnt from the international studies that Betts and Huet (2023) brought together in *Bridging the Creative Arts Therapies and Arts in Health.*

Three initiatives are particularly salient to this provocation:

Developing a Continuum of Practice

Moss (2008) laid the foundation for a Continuum of Practice whereby the work of both CPs and CATs can be viewed along a continuum from institutional care in hospitals and clinics with CATs at the clinical end to CPs at the community end. This continuum 'can be conceptualised as ranging from a clinical focus at one end of the spectrum to a broad public health focus at the other end' (Lambert, Lee and Sonke 2023 p.66). The development of a Continuum of Practice is exemplified by the Creative Forces® arts for injured veterans programme, which, as Vaudreuil, Blumenfeld and Walker (2023) point out, also benefits from an integrated R&D (research and development) building capacity that supports the development of both CPs and CATs. Neither group is disenfranchised, as the contribution of both groups is valued and they both benefit from being aware of and linked into each other's practice.

Joining up the education and training of practitioners

Arts in health work in the USA is led by the National Organization for Arts in Health (NOAH), which, in a leadership summit, proposed the framework for a long-term coalition of stakeholders to address the future of arts in health in the USA in order to:

> ...build capacity for future research, educational efforts, and workforce and resource development focusing on arts and humanities' role in supporting an individual's health and wellbeing and the community engagement needed to secure infrastructure across the health and wellbeing continuum. (NOAH 2018 p.1)

Integrated arts and health pathways

The Creative Forces® project (Vaudreuil *et al.* 2023) also shows how pathways and systems can be organised in ways that facilitate access to arts therapy and arts in health and meet the needs of the 'the whole person' (an injured veteran) by making a range of expertise available *at different stages of illness and recovery*. Boundaries must be malleable, and pathways to appropriate support and services, accessible and non-linear. Whilst no similar structured pathways exist in the UK, there is scope to include arts and health in NHS care pathways, for example in the Dementia Care Pathway (Royal College of Psychiatrists 2025), specifically in person-centred post-diagnosis support when most people who are diagnosed in memory clinics continue to live in their own home. These include people with lived experience of the condition supported by family carers who are vital in meeting the needs of their loved ones and, as Talbot (2022) argues, also in relation to the importance of meaningful occupation and social engagement.

Next steps in the UK
Creating a continuum of arts and health practice

Creative dialogue and collaboration between CPs, CATs and other stakeholders will begin to dismantle artificial 'professional silos' (Betts and Huet 2023). A Continuum of Practice that enables each group to be represented, that highlights the reciprocity and democratic value in the idea, with therapy handing over to community arts and vice versa, within the context of creative arts in health. In practice, this means a person being treated at one instance by a CAT, over time can be referred into a community based creative health initiative run by a CP and vice versa. In the UK, the development of a Continuum of Arts in Health practice will involve research and consultation with key stakeholders including the NHS, HCPC and other professional bodies. CHWA and NCCH are well placed to champion this work especially since its inception in 2020 CHWA has promoted dialogue between CATs and CPs and arts, health and wellbeing organisations, and NCCH is leading macro level initiatives especially in primary and community care.

Workforce development: education and training for arts in health practice

Despite considerable gaps in education, training and continuing professional development (CPD) for many CPs and others working in arts in health (see Chapter 15), an expansion of the arts in health workforce is taking place, notwithstanding the silos of creative arts practice that have their roots in separate education and training whence one group of students (CATs) qualify as professionals and others do not. New arts and health jobs, as well as CPs seeking degrees, are also driving demand for new courses. In these, and CAT courses, the inclusion of modules about the creative arts practice landscape, skills and knowledge, and the roles and relationships of CATs and CPs, could also help facilitate more awareness raising, dialogue and collaboration. Building blocks are being put in place by encouraging CPs and CATS to come together in different contexts to share their knowledge and skills as part of professional development (Hume 2023).

Creating arts, health and wellbeing care pathways

Integrating the arts into clinical care pathways would help meet unmet needs, especially at points where there are often gaps in service continuity. For example, many people diagnosed with dementia at a memory clinic often become aware of a gap in community support after returning home following their diagnosis. Here, properly funded social prescribing of creative arts may meet their needs for meaningful occupation and social engagement. Another example is post-discharge, as arts-in-hospital patient engagement usually ceases at a point when many vulnerable older people are at risk of readmission. One model that deserves further piloting is Bristol Southmead Hospital's 'Fresh Arts on Referral' (Willis Newson 2019) whereby patients receive CP support on their return home from hospital. Replicating this approach and comparing health outcomes and other measures with standard practice would be worthwhile.

Support for practitioners and organisations providing supervision and mentoring

As noted here and in Chapters 15 and 17, several organisations have begun providing resources and support that reduce practitioner isolation (especially CPs) and contribute to workforce development. CATs are now widely involved in mentoring, supervising and evaluating arts and health projects in London and supervising individual CPs, enabling them to develop their skills in reflective practices and improving the quality of care provided (Sandford and Gilluley 2021). These developments, however, are individual initiatives, sporadic and unlikely to deliver even coverage across the UK unless funding is made available.

Implications

Systems change does not take place without disruption of the status quo. Increased collaboration between CATs and CPs highlights overarching areas of tension (Moss 2016) that need to be addressed, including: '[p]rofessional insecurities, lack of clear definition of roles and professional boundaries and competition for funding between different arts practitioners in the field' (*ibid.* p.7). These are likely to act as a brake to developing joint projects involving CATs and CPs.

Furthermore, discussions with CATs suggest that it may be difficult for them, their employers and professional bodies to establish and agree the basis on which they might be available to help develop and support CPs through dialogue, mentoring, supervision, etc. Macro-level discussions also need to include CAT professional bodies and universities, since course providers skilling up CPs may well enhance their status and make them more attractive to project funders and perhaps also service commissioners and providers. Given their rates of pay are considerably lower than CATs, this would be contentious for CATs; however, the fifth of the five recommendations made by the Baring Foundation's report *Creatively Minded and the NHS* is that 'Mental Health Trusts should explore how Creative Arts Therapists and Participatory Artists can most productively share their differing skills and support each other to the benefit of patients' (Cutler 2021 p.65).

Conclusion

This positive provocation makes the case for more creative dialogue and collaboration between the creative arts in health and wellbeing and creative arts therapy. Evidence of the benefits of arts in health and wellbeing for meeting psychological and social need is driving demand for creative arts, especially for people living with dementia and their carers. The Covid-19 pandemic highlighted the value of arts engaging in health and wellbeing with different populations and the advantages of partnership working on arts in health practice (Chapple *et al.* 2023). The NHS backed further expansion of social prescribing, and Creative Health Associates (CHAs) are now working with commissioning groups and local integrated care systems in England. CHAs are professionals who promote creative health within the NHS and are hosted by Integrated Care Boards in each region in England. They facilitate the integration of creative activities in healthcare. In addition, the inclusion of arts and culture in Wales (The Well-Being of Future Generations/Wales Act) has become a significant priority for the Welsh Government, with culture central to national identity and crucial to individual and community wellbeing (Welsh Government 2024).

Despite similarities and differences, obstacles to creative dialogue and collaboration remain between CATs and CPs. There are signs this is changing, however, and we would wholeheartedly support this move, as working together in practitioner support, supervision and mentoring is crucial to developing a high-quality arts and health workforce and making the most of limited funds. Creative dialogue and collaboration are essential for developing a Continuum of Practice, joining up the education and training of practitioners and supporting integrated arts and healthcare pathways for people living with dementia, whilst also addressing the implications.

There are lessons to be learnt about strategic partnerships between arts, health and social care on other stages, including internationally, where arts in health collaboration has come about because organisations have been willing to embrace complexity and interconnectedness, work across organisational boundaries and build active partnerships as part of systems change. A final call then to readers to help realise Moss's 'New Paradigm' (2016) and rally around Vaudreuil *et al.*'s (2023) call for '[b]uilding a Clinic to Community Continuum through the Arts' (p.107) to help improve national health and wellbeing as we move inexorably into the middle of the 21st century.

Acknowledgements

With thanks to Marina Benini, Dr Mary Coaten, Fergus Early OBE, Emily Hoffman, Antigone Ikkos, Dr Steven Michael OBE, Lois Pignéguy, Dr Allison Singer, Jacqui Terry-Schuhmann, Helen Webster and Professors Hilary Moss and Helen Payne for supporting the creation of this chapter.

References

Armstrong, M., Aker, N., Pushpa, N., Walters K., *et al.* (2022) 'Trust and inclusion during the Covid-19 pandemic: Perspectives from Black and South Asian people living with dementia and their carers in the UK.' *International Journal of Geriatric Psychiatry* 37, 3, 1–13.

Betts, D. and Huet, V. (eds) (2023) *Bridging the Creative Arts Therapies and Arts in Health: Toward Inspirational Practice*. London: Jessica Kingsley Publishers.

Bradbury, A., Warran, K., Mak, H. W. and Fancourt, D. (2021) *The Role of the Arts During the COVID-19 Pandemic*. London: UCL.

Chapple, M., Anisimovich, A., Worsley, J., Watkins, M., Billington, J. and Balabanova, E. (2023) 'Come together: The importance of arts and cultural engagement within the Liverpool City Region throughout the COVID-19 lockdown periods.' *Frontiers in Psychology* 13, 1011771.

Cutler, B. (2021) *Creatively Minded and the NHS*. London: The Baring Foundation. https://cdn. baringfoundation.org.uk/wp-content/uploads/BF_Creatively-minded-the-NHS_WEB.pdf

Dow, R., Warran, K., Letrondo, P. and Fancourt, D. (2023) 'The arts in public health policy: Progress and opportunities.' *The Lancet Public Health* 8, 2, e155–e160.

Heddon, D., O'Neill, M., Rose, M., Qualmann, C. and Wilson, H. (2021) *Walking Publics, Walking Arts*. Glasgow: University of Glasgow. https://walkcreate.gla.ac.uk

Hume, V. (2023) 'Mutual Support? What Do the Creative Arts Therapies and Creativity and Culture for Health and Well-Being Bring to Each Other?' In D. Betts and V. Huet (2023) (eds) *Bridging the Creative Arts Therapies and Arts in Health: Toward Inspirational Practice*. London: Jessica Kingsley Publishers.

Lambert, P., Lee, J. and Sonke, L. (2023) 'Educating Artists and Administrators to Engage the Arts in Health and Well-Being in Healthcare and Community Settings.' In D. Betts and V. Huet (2023) (eds) *Bridging the Creative Arts Therapies and Arts in Health: Toward Inspirational Practice*. London: Jessica Kingsley Publishers.

Moss, H. (2008) 'Reflections on Music Therapy and Arts in Health.' *British Journal of Music Therapy 22*, 2, 84–87.

Moss, H. (2016) 'Arts and health: A new paradigm.' *Voices: A World Forum for Music Therapy 16*, 3.

NOAH (National Organization for Arts in Health) (2017) *Arts, Health, and Wellbeing in America*. San Diego, CA: Author.

NOAH (National Organization for Arts in Health) (2018) *Addressing the Future of Arts in Health in America*. San Diego, CA: Author.

NCCH and APPG AHW (National Centre for Creative Health and the All-Party Parliamentary Group on Arts, Health, and Wellbeing) (2023) *Creative Health Review: How Policy Can Embrace Creative Health*. https://ncch.org.uk/creative-health-review

NHS (2019) *The NHS Long Term Plan*. www.longtermplan.nhs.uk/wp-content/uploads/2019/08/nhs-long-term-plan-version-1.2.pdf

NHS England (2020) Workforce Training and Education – Art, Drama and Music Therapists under Allied Health Professional Workforce Reform Priorities (2020–2021). www.hee.nhs.uk/our-work/allied-health-professions/art-drama-music-therapists

Percy-Smith, B., Bailey, R., Stenberg, N., Booth-Kurpnieks, C. *et al.* (2024) *Creative Health in Communities: Supporting People to Live Well in West Yorkshire*. https://research.hud.ac.uk/media/assets/photo/art/temporarycontemporary/Creative-Health-in-Communities-FinalMarch24.pdf

Royal College of Psychiatrists (2025) Dementia pathway. www.rcpsych.ac.uk/improving-care/nccmh/service-design-and-development/dementia

Sandford, S. and Gilluley, P. (2021) 'The East London Foundation Trust.' In B. Cutler (2021) (ed.) *Creatively Minded and the NHS*. London: The Baring Foundation. https://cdn.baring-foundation.org.uk/wp-content/uploads/BF_Creatively-minded-the-NHS_WEB.pdf

Sheffield Hallam University (2024) New model to embed arts and creative activities in hospitals. www.shu.ac.uk/news/all-articles/latest-news/creative-health-boards

Talbot, M. (2022) 'The Practical Realities of Caring for a Loved One with Dementia.' In I. Parker, R. Coaten and M. Hopfenbeck (eds) *The Practical Handbook of Living with Dementia*. Monmouth: PCCS Books.

Vaudreuil, R., Blumenfeld, H. and Walker, M. (2023) 'Creative Forces®: The Continuum of Clinical Creative Arts Therapies to Community Arts Engagement for Military-Connected Populations.' In D. Betts and V. Huet (2023) (eds) *Bridging the Creative Arts Therapies and Arts in Health: Toward Inspirational Practice*. London: Jessica Kingsley Publishers.

Well-Being of Future Generations (Wales) Act (2015) www.futuregenerations.wales/about-us/future-generations-act

Welsh Government (2024) *Consultation on the Draft Priorities for Culture in Wales 2024–2030*. Cardiff: Welsh Government.

Willis Newson (2019) *Fresh Arts on Referral Evaluation: Summary Document*. Bristol: Willis Newson. www.willisnewson.co.uk/assets/files/fresh-arts-on-referral-evaluation-doc-260319.pdf

Wiltshire, K. and Prescott, D. (2023) 'Create, connect, unwind: A creative response to the pandemic for NHS staff well-being.' *Journal of Applied Arts and Health 14*, 2, 257–269.

CHAPTER 19

Working with People Living with Dementia

Creative Arts Practice in the Next Decade and Beyond

Maria Pasiecznik Parsons and Richard Coaten

Aim and context

This practice handbook has equipped Creative Health Practitioners (CHPs), especially Creative Practitioners (CPs) and Creative Arts Therapists (CATs) who work with people living with dementia, with an understanding of values, knowledge and skills for practice. We hope that it has also raised awareness of creative arts for dementia and its contribution to the creative health agenda amongst other relevant stakeholders, including commissioners, managers and funders.

Reflecting on now and the next decade, we can see threads running throughout the handbook. How, where and in what ways can these threads coalesce and be woven together into a coherent whole that can strengthen creative arts for dementia and foster its growth?

For this reason, in this last chapter, we revisit vibrant and inspirational threads – art forms and approaches – used by our co-authors to connect with and relate to people living with dementia. Their work showcases the diversity of practice in this field that we hope will attract interest from other practitioners and those contemplating this work. To build on this interest, one important thread is the need to make more training and professional development available to grow the creative health workforce (see Chapters 14, 15, 17 and 18) and to expand support for practitioners, especially freelancers (see Chapter 17), to ensure a workforce fit for the future, given the increasing prevalence of dementia in the UK and rising demand for support and services amongst individuals and families.

In several places, we acknowledge that demographic change is a driver in population ageing: a longer old age but with increased risk of dementia. Globally, too, needs are increasing; current projections are that 78 million people will be living with the condition in 2030 and 139 million in 2050, with prevalence rising fastest in low- to middle-income countries in 'the global south' including BRICS countries such as China and India (Long, Benoist and Weidner 2023). Many of these societies have substantial populations of younger people and older people, between whom close relationships are traditionally facilitated, but economic change is disrupting communities. In the UK, more opportunities for cross-generational contact need to be developed (Burke 2024). Creative arts are an excellent medium for facilitating intergenerational relationships between people living with dementia and children and young people (Jenkins, Farrer and Aujla 2021).

The person comes first is a thread that emerges from Chapter 1 and is taken up in Chapter 2, which explicates many of the key concepts of personhood, person-centred approaches and values (Kitwood 1997) that underpin good practice in arts and dementia. From there, we are aware of these concepts being a constant thread, particularly in supporting the selfhood of the person living with dementia, which is ultimately bound up with relationships and social interactions that involve art and poetry in Chapter 3, music in Chapter 4 and dance in Chapter 5. In Chapter 6, a poet describes how she prepares and presents a range of poems that she uses to relate to participants who create beautiful rhymes, often with strong rhythms in which we glimpse sensual, embodied and unconscious dimensions of the emotional self.

Chapters 9 and 10 acknowledge that maintaining the personhood of care home residents and hospital patients in busy environments challenges not only health and care staff but also CPs. CPs are more transient care partners who seek to build caring and trusting relationships despite coming onto wards or into care home lounges once weekly. Almost half a million people live in residential and care homes, of whom 70% have dementia (Care Home and Nursing Home Information and Advice 2025). Chapter 9 highlights the work of arts providers, who enable older, frailer residents to engage in arts and activities. The employment of CPs is valued but sporadic, given the staffing and cost pressures experienced by care home providers. Chapter 10 describes the wide-ranging creative arts 'palette' of a hospital arts manager. Here, CPs work with multidisciplinary staff, particularly nurses, whose support is crucial in getting to know patients and working in ways that take account of health cultures, protocols and processes.

Another (shorter) thread is our UK, somewhat England-centric, focus on creative arts for dementia and a definition framed in a Western cultural tradition, one that privileges purposeful engagement and structured activities. Nevertheless, we recognise the value of everyday creativity – arts and cultural activities undertaken in day-to-day life (not for a health purpose per se but having a secondary benefit for health). In groups, communities and cultures, both in the UK and globally, people living with dementia enjoy leisure activities – often music or connecting with nature – as well as taking part in community life, cultural activities, spiritual practices or activities associated with religious observance.

The growing diversity of our society makes it imperative for practice to be inclusive. As a community, we need to address the marginalisation of people from Black and Minority Ethnic communities as participants in creative arts for dementia and to support greater diversity of CHPs both now and in the future. Such inclusion also needs to support the development of socially and culturally appropriate resources that promote cultural forms of expression (Kaimal and Arslanbek 2020). Chapter 8 offers good practice in this respect. A museum team that developed the House of Memories (HoM) reminiscence app went on to co-produce a customised HoM Yemeni elders app with members of the Yemeni community. The app includes socially and culturally relevant memories for older people, including those living with dementia. More information can be found at: www.liverpoolmuseums.org.uk/house-of-memories/connecting-yemeni-elders-heritage.

Beyond noting the barriers to accessing culturally competent support, there is little in the way of a 'rainbow thread' in this handbook. The voices of people living with dementia and their care partners and supporters who identify as LGBTQ+ have become more prominent through the activism of self-organised groups, including a Community Interest Company (CIC) (Parish and Bond 2023). The *Journal of Dementia Care* special issue on equality, diversity and inclusion provides an important grounding for CATs and CPs in diverse communities and their responses to dementia (Whitman and Truswell 2023).

Creating 'wholes' out of fragments

Much of what we do as practitioners is to work with fragments of memories, stories, songs, feelings and sensations (Coaten 2001). It is what we do with whatever we are given, together with how we notice, respond to and celebrate the fragments, that matters. I refer, very briefly, to Laurie, who convincingly uses the 'three Cs of RBC (Rapport Based Communication)' (Laurie 2022 p.171). First, to see the 'offer' that the person is giving to us, either verbally or non-verbally; second, to 'copy'; then, to 'celebrate' it. In celebrating it, we give back to the person something of their essence, which they have communicated (to us). In the fundamentally relational and creative space that we practise in, this two-way process is of immense importance in helping people living with the condition to know they still have much to give, share and be valued for. The valuing in itself brings a sense of coherence, and the contents of this handbook attest to these facts.

The idea of celebration, coupled with a strong message of hope, is contained in Taylor, Peterson and Poet's powerful description in Chapter 7 of how the award-winning play *Maggie May* was co-created by people living with dementia. They were involved in all stages of its devising, rehearsal and performance. It gave to the audience, as the authors describe, not only a 'balanced story of adapting and coping' but also a clear message about 'what's possible when we co-create and value voices that are less often part of the conversation'. The play also broke new ground by moving away from a tragedy narrative, inviting people to think differently about dementia, while weaving threads together theatrically into an emotionally moving and coherent whole. A focus on learning from each other's experiences of living with the condition and finding solutions through dialogue to the many production challenges were also key to the process. This is echoed by Amanze, who says in Chapter 12, 'Art has made me visible and given me a voice where I had no voice.' These threads of finding a voice, becoming visible and feeling valued, together with a sense of belonging, are echoed throughout the chapters in respect of practice and underpinning research.

These are powerful forward-looking messages of empowerment. We must take them into account now and in the future, given our socio-economic challenges, including climate change. They give hope, as they are also, metaphorically speaking, strengthened by the warp and the weft of their construction: the vertical and horizontal structures used in the weaving process. Full of hope are the 'beautiful garments' created from the relationship between the two that weaves them together. In this context, we have the vertical threads or structures of the arts practices themselves but without the weft or the horizontal and relational aspects that are encompassed by the values governing our work, including person-centred and relationship-centred care (Nolan, Keady and Aveyard 2001), that reinforce the 'how' of what we do. The two act in synchrony to enable us to feel that participation has meaning, gives joy and offers emotional interpersonal reassurance.

Family carers

All over the world, family carers are the cornerstone of care for loved ones living with dementia and the whole foundation in many low-income countries where statutory support is underdeveloped.

To think, feel, sense and intuit how best to help loved ones makes sense of what often appears to be a conundrum, for example, having to accept that a driving licence has to be taken away by a government agency. Here, a sense of independence, strongly attached to value, impacts on self-esteem and identity. Other losses are experienced too of course, and the challenges faced by a creative carer in managing and supporting their loved one to accept these losses or otherwise can be considerable (see Chapter 2). The handbook includes examples of good practice in meeting family carers' needs, through positive and inclusive practice of musical composition (see Chapter 4) and empowerment through dance (see Chapter 5) and performance (see Chapter 11). However, given increasing demands on family carers, we need to learn and understand how creative arts might best provide emotional, physical, psychological and spiritual support, particularly for community-dwelling family carers. We must learn from 'The Mountains I Still Climb', in Amanze and Truswell (see Chapter 12) and specifically the words:

> *And if you can't hear me*
> *When I'm calling*
> *How you gonna know*
> *That I'm falling?*
> (AMANZE 2019)

Amanze wrote these words about himself, but in our opinion, they also resonate strongly for family carers. This is as much as anything a moral and economic imperative to support family carers that also is an important aspect of social justice. For individuals and families in the UK bear the largest burden of the total costs of dementia care – forecasted in 2024 as £42 billion, with 50% borne by individuals and families. This is estimated to rise to 63% of the forecasted £90.1 billion total costs by 2040 (Alzheimer's Society and Carnall Farrar 2024). Present and future family carers 'save' the NHS and local councils money in their care budgets. As Amanze also said in Chapter 12 about his own experience, which can be transposed across to the family carer, he is not just 'a vehicle or item' on someone else's agenda, like a box that must be ticked. Each family carer journey is unique, as is the journey of everyone living with the condition. Their needs are different, as evidenced by an arts therapist running a creative arts group for older people living with dementia (see Chapter 17). She was hopeful that family carers might be able to stay and take part. The vast majority were grateful for the offer but indicated they instead needed these two hours for respite.

Embodied practice

A phrase from Chapter 11, from Allegranti's work on *Moving Kinship* hubs – 'a newly embodied way of relating must be found for all; if not, the impact of a dementia diagnosis and way of life will be a traumatising legacy' – has been selected by Richard, a dance and movement psychotherapist, as fundamental to his practice going forward. The thinking needs unravelling in this uncompromising statement. However, while the argument is complex, it centres on what is meant by an 'embodied way of relating', using practices that are embodied and what happens if we don't practise in these ways.

The word 'embodiment' that is at the heart of embodied practices is loaded with many assumptions, but Allegranti (see Chapter 11) and Brierley (see Chapter 5) are articulate and comprehensive in their different perspectives of what working in embodied ways means. We are consciously trying to become aware of the physical, affective and complex ways that we experience ourselves in our bodies. It means being attentive to how we communicate non-verbally, especially where cognitive processing is poor. Can we sense the strong relationship between body language and emotional expression, sometimes the only way people can express themselves? Are we alert to how our presence and our own movement language might be perceived by others? How do we use and modulate the tonal qualities and volume in our voices to express a sense of enabling the person to feel heard and met? When we movers, DMPs and CATs, speak of 'mirroring' (Levy 2015) a person, what do we mean? Why is it so important that when we are alongside people using this approach, it helps them to feel safe and to calm them if they are upset?

We work with the language of the body because we all exist in one – we all have one, but not everyone is even aware of, let alone appreciates, the subtle skill sets possessed by dancers, CATs and somatic movement educators. These skill sets are arguably essential to what current dementia researchers are telling us about the importance of staying physically active for our mental and physical health (Pope *et al.* 2019). As Brierley says in Chapter 5, 'carers share how dance supports relaxation and shifts mood when they are exhausted or at "the end of their tether"', while another 'identifies how sessions offer her "emotional support" and "time thinking about my own body"' and a third experiences being 'less stressed at the end of the sessions, much calmer and able to cope'. However, where does this leave the vexing aspect of a 'traumatising legacy' if embodied practices are not a part of the practitioner's lexicon? The key aspect of Allegranti's argument appears in relation to the importance of how, in what can be described as a sociological and analytic framework, intersectionality (Crenshaw 1989) manifests in the care of people living with dementia and creative arts practice. To what extent are we, as CHPs or CATs, aware of our own unique combinations of privilege and disadvantage that interact and combine? For these, as described by Allegranti in Chapter 11, potentially impact hugely on what we do in our work. Our gender, our race, our ethnicity, our sexual orientation, our disability and our societal class are enmeshed in the ways in which we practise our craft. There is no escaping them, as they are the elements that have made us uniquely who and how we are.

However, in working with vulnerable adults living with dementia and their professional and family carers, we risk a 'traumatising legacy' if we are not fully aware of how these qualities in practice may manifest. There can be prejudices, as well as advantages, that can add to or take away from how people with the condition are already discriminated against in relation to the challenges they already have to deal with. This is not just about CHPs and CATs learning how to work with a great deal more awareness of intersectionality. It is about the whole dementia care workforce taking it seriously and receiving training in intersectionality as well. Going forward, embodied practices and intersectionality should go hand in hand. Awareness of the embodied practices alerts all practitioners to the importance of working with and through the 'body'. Acknowledging intersectionality ensures that we do not prejudice our work by failing to address the wider contexts within which we work that encompass our personal biases. As CHPs and CATS of whatever art form, we would do well to take these two key elements into what we do in future.

The UK context in which creative arts for dementia takes place is characterised by significant fiscal pressures in health and social care and in arts and culture, and is likely to remain so in the near future. However, effective delivery of social prescribing (SP) is one component of a multidisciplinary and integrated approach to health and wellbeing across the lifespan being developed by the NHS and supported by creative health. Chapter 13 describes the experience of an arts organisation that has strong roots in the community and is involved in the SP of arts and health activities in collaboration with health/social care and voluntary sector partners. The chapter includes a short literature review that suggests the evidence for SP is promising but more research is needed to understand specific mechanisms contributing to participants' outcomes and longitudinal effects of participation. In Chapter 17 we have reported on both the rewards and challenges of working freelance in this sector. The post-COVID-19 recovery of creative arts for dementia has been slow and steady, but funding across arts, health and social care will remain very tight for the foreseeable future (HM Government 2025). Nevertheless, such evidence contributes to the achievement of one of the goals of creative health: to become an embedded and valued part of health and care systems and available to all.

We close by drawing together some of the threads of good practice in creative arts for dementia, which were requested by many members of our community at the inception of the project to develop a practice handbook and which are demonstrated throughout:

- an understanding of dementia
- person-centred approaches and values
- ethical considerations (including those informed by intersectionality)
- the creative process
- the use of embodied practices
- co-creation and co-production
- providing a safe and supportive environment
- making, sustaining and ending relationships
- communication, improvisation and providing opportunities for self-expression, self-identity, imagination, creativity, enjoyment, pleasure and celebration
- varying a session tempo between active and quiet
- fostering social connections and reciprocity
- collaboration with staff and families
- meeting needs for personal and professional development
- self-care and support.

As Community Practitioners and Creative Arts Therapists, we always seek to improve the quality of life for people with lived experience of dementia and their caregivers. We know that we can do this work well by paying attention to the list above, which summarises some of what makes practice 'good'.

However, in the face of many challenges to the work we do, globally, environmentally, economically and socially and psychologically, we end this handbook by asking readers to connect and collaborate whenever and wherever they can.

Both organisational collaboration and working together as a community of practice are key to creative health that can contribute significantly to national government plans and policies that prioritise helping individuals, families and services to focus on prevention and managing specific conditions, particularly in primary care and at the community (place based) level.

At the strategic level, we have flagged the need for partnership between statutory, voluntary and commercial sectors through mechanisms such as SP and effective joint working between CHPs and staff in cultural venues, NHS hospital trusts, care homes, meeting centres and schools. Many of the chapters show the field of practice is replete with 'project-based, short-term work' but we highlight examples of collaboration underpinned by joint funding/resourcing, facilitating more sustainable arts for dementia work. More are needed.

However, if we are to meet the needs of more individuals and family carers needing our services going forward, whilst resources become increasingly stretched and cuts continue to be made across arts, health and social care funding, we need to take collective action. To grow peer networks, to share and support each other through, for example, special interest groups of dancers or musicians, to offer and exchange resources and become active in the Culture, Health and Wellbeing Alliance, or in other national networks.

Let's keep making a difference to people's lives – leaving the last words about why we do this to Ronald Amanze, who in Chapter 12 tells us what this work really means for him:

> The biggest thing that keeps me going is creative expression through art. Art makes me breathe. It helps me breathe without embarrassment. It helps me reflect on life without regret. It makes me gravitate towards beautiful conversations. It really works for me.

References

Alzheimer's Society and Carnall Farrar (2024) *The Economic Impact of Dementia*. Alzheimer's Society: London. www.carnallfarrar.com/wp-content/uploads/2024/06/The-economic-impact-of-dementia-CF.pdf

Amanze, R. (2019) 'The Mountains I Still Climb.' Dementia Diaries with Ronald Amanze. https://dementiadiaries.org/entry/10124/the-mountains-i-still-climb

Burke, S. (2024) *Changing Britain for All Ages: Ten Intergenerational Steps Towards Shared Futures*. Wivenhoe: United for All Ages. www.unitedforallages.com/_files/ugd/98d289_ba7348f-0fa50400a9a6aa1dd63d92af8.pdf

Care Home and Nursing Home Information and Advice (2025) Care home facts & stats: settings, population & workforce. www.carehome.co.uk/advice/care-home-stats-number-of-settings-population-workforce

Coaten, R. (2001) 'Exploring reminiscence through dance and movement.' *Journal of Dementia Care* 9, 5, 19–22.

Crenshaw, K. (1989) 'Demarginalizing the intersection of race and sex: A Black feminist critique of antidiscrimination doctrine, feminist theory and antiracist politics.' *University of Chicago Legal Forum* 139, 139–168.

HM Government (2025) Treasury Spending Review June 2025. www.gov.uk/government/publications/spending-review-2025-document/spending-review-2025-html

Jenkins, L. K., Farrer, R. and Aujla, I. J. (2021) 'Understanding the impact of an intergenerational arts and health project: A study into the psychological well-being of participants, carers and artists.' *Public Health* 194, 121–126.

Kaimal, G. and Arslanbek, A. (2020) 'Indigenous and traditional visual artistic practices: implications for art therapy clinical practice and research.' *Frontiers in Psychology* 11, 1320.

Kitwood, T. (1997) *Dementia Reconsidered: The Person Comes First*. Buckingham: Open University Press.

Laurie, M. (2022) 'Rapport-Based Communication: A Practical Approach to Social Inclusion and Mutual Wellbeing.' In I. Parker, R. Coaten and M. Hopfenbeck (eds) *The Practical Handbook of Living with Dementia*. Monmouth: PCCS Books.

Levy, F. (2015) *Dance Movement Therapy a Healing Art*. Revised edition. Baltimore, MD: Amer Alliance for Health Physical.

Long, S., Benoist, C. and Weidner, W. (2023) *World Alzheimer Report. Reducing Dementia Risk: Never Too Early, Never Too Late*. London: Alzheimer's Disease International. www.alzint.org/u/World-Alzheimer-Report-2023.pdf

Nolan, M., Keady, J. and Aveyard, B. (2001) 'Relationship-centred care is the next logical step.' *British Journal of Nursing* 10, 12, 757.

Parish, M. and Bond, J. A. (2023) 'Queering up dementia care: The next steps.' *Journal of Dementia Care 31*, 5, 33–35.

Pope, J., Helwig, K., Morrison, S., Estep, A., Caswell, S., Ambegaonkar, J. and Cortes, N. (2019) 'Multifactorial exercise and dance-based interventions are effective in reducing falls risk in community-dwelling older adults: a comparison study.' *Gait and Posture 70*, 370–375.

Whitman, L. and Truswell, D. (2023) 'Equality, diversity and inclusion: A special issue.' *Journal of Dementia Care 31*, 5. https://journalofdementiacare.co.uk/wp-content/uploads/2023/10/JDCSEPT23.pdf

Subject Index

Author Index